# anatomy of
# RUNNING

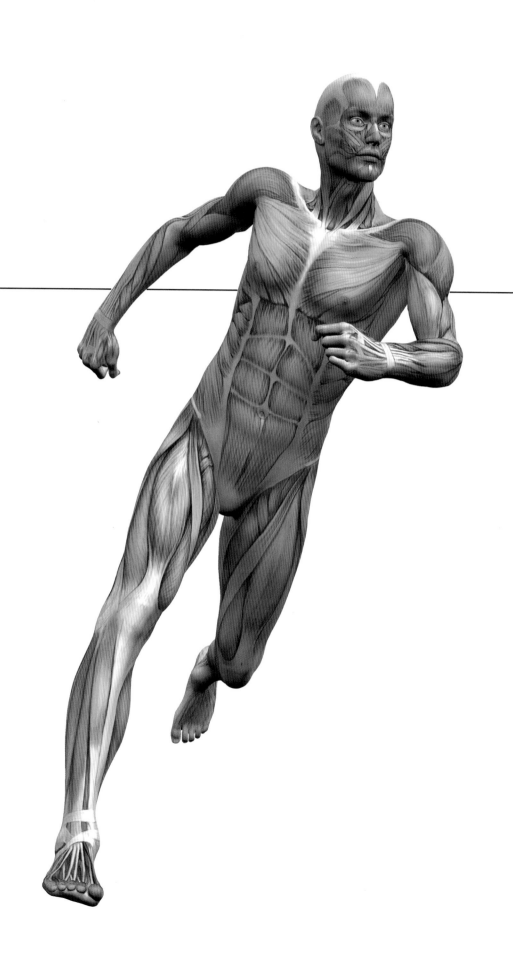

# anatomy of
# RUNNING

Philip Striano, DC

FIREFLY BOOKS

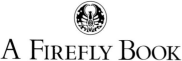

# A FIREFLY BOOK

Published by Firefly Books Ltd. 2013

Copyright © 2013 Moseley Road Inc.

First printing

**Publisher Cataloging-in-Publication Data (U.S.)**
A CIP record for this title is available from Library of Congress

**Library and Archives Canada Cataloguing in Publication**
A CIP record for this title is available from Library and Archives Canada

Published in the United States by
Firefly Books (U.S.) Inc.
P.O. Box 1338, Ellicott Station
Buffalo, New York  14205

Published in Canada by
Firefly Books Ltd.
50 Staples Avenue, Unit 1
Richmond Hill, Ontario  L4B 0A7

Printed in China

*Anatomy of Running* was developed by:
Moseley Road Inc.
123 Main Street
Irvington, New York 10533

**Moseley Road Inc.**
President: Sean Moore
General Manager: Karen Prince

Project Editor/Designer: Lisa Purcell

Production Designers: Terasa Bernard, Adam Moore

Photographer: Jonathan Conklin Photography, Inc.

Models: Nicolay Alexandrov, Sara Blowers

# CONTENTS

# CONTENTS continued

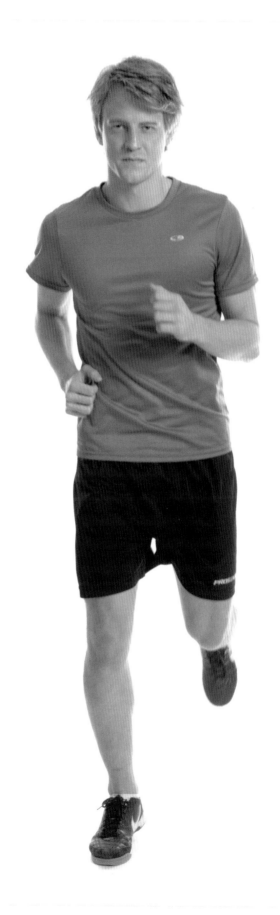

# INTRODUCTION:
# WHY RUN?

Running and jogging are among the most popular recreational sports in the world. So why do so many people from diverse backgrounds choose to run? Of course, each individual has unique motivations, but there are several goals shared by many runners, from a desire to lose weight to a need to lower blood pressure and strengthen the heart.

Running is also a versatile way to get fit—you can run just about anytime and anywhere, and it is a relatively inexpensive sport. It doesn't require pricey health club memberships or personal training fees. With little more than the right pair of shoes, anyone of just about any age and fitness level can start a running regimen. Yet, as with any physical activity, there is a right way and a wrong way to run—don't expect to just lace up your running shoes and hit the pavement. You should also prepare for and augment your running routine with stretches and exercises geared to warming you up before a run and cooling you down after it, and perform strengthening exercises that target the key muscles used in running. Take the time to learn how to run right, using the guidelines found in the following pages.

# YOUR RUNNING ROUTINE

Most of us are aware that running is a great way to lose weight and to get leaner and stronger, but its benefits are so much more than skin deep. Running is not just about improving your appearance, in fact, running is more about improving your overall health and allowing your body to perform at its highest levels.

These are some of the most common reasons for running and the benefits you'll receive:

### Burns calories
Running burns about 100 calories per hour (the more you weigh the more calories you'll burn), so weight loss is a prime incentive for many beginner runners, and weight maintenance for those who run regularly.

### Increases lean body mass
Your lean body mass is made up of everything in your body besides fat, including your

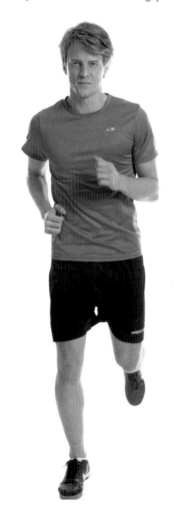

organs, blood, skin, bones, and muscles. In general, a lower fat-to-muscle ratio is healthier. Running reduces fat and thereby lowers your fat-to-muscle ratio.

### Increases VO$_2$ max
Your VO$_2$ max, or maximal oxygen consumption, is generally the amount of oxygen your body can transport and use during incremental exercise. Peak oxygen uptake equals peak physical condition—increasing your VO$_2$ max allows you to perform at your best.

### Regulates cholesterol levels
Regular running can help you regulate cholesterol levels, lowering the "bad" LDL cholesterol levels, while increasing the "good" HDL levels.

### Increases bone density
Weight-bearing exercise, such as running, increases bone density—the measurement of the mineral content inside your bones—which helps protect you from osteoporosis-related fractures.

### Improves psychological health
The psychological benefits of running are many: with its endorphin-boosting power, running decreases stress and increases confidence. Running allows you to easily set—and meet—tangible goals, which makes you feel good about yourself. It also improves your self-image; the physical changes you

see in the mirror will give your self-esteem a boost and provide you with the incentive to stick to your running regimen.

## HOW TO GET STARTED

Ease into a running routine. You want to incrementally build your strength and endurance; as your muscles and cardiovascular system adapt, you can slowly begin to build on your increased capacity. Taking it slow will help you prevent injury and avoid frustration.

Before beginning any exercise regimen, check with your primary care physician to determine whether you are healthy enough to run or have any special considerations that you need to allow for within your running routine.

### Warming Up and Cooling Down

To get the most from your run, take the time to warm up before you set out and cool down when you stop.

Proper stretching leads to better performance and should be a key component

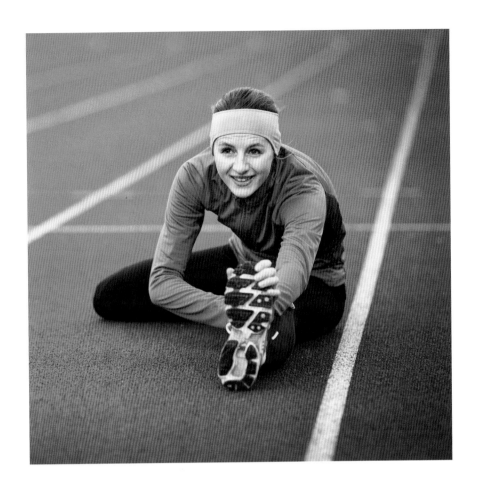

of both your pre-run routine and your post-run cool-down. Never stretch cold muscles, which are more prone to injury. To warm up before a pre-run stretch, take just 5 minutes to run in place, jump rope, or do a few push-ups—any activity that gets the heart pumping and blood flowing into muscles. After your run, again take a few minutes to perform some stretching exercises.

### Take It Slowly

Once you are ready to begin, start by walking 20 minutes three times a week. Do not walk on consecutive days—allow your body to recover between walking sessions.

During the second week, if you feel fine physically, combine walking and running for 20 minutes on three nonconsecutive

### BORN TO RUN

Running may be one of the most natural forms of exercises you can choose. Scientific evidence suggests that the human body evolved quite literally to run—and to run over long distances. Our flexible leg and foot ligaments and tendons act like springs, and our narrow midsections allow us to swing our arms and keep us from weaving off a trail. A highly developed sense of balance keeps us stable while on the move. Even our toes are made for running—they are relatively short compared to our ape relatives', and our big toes are straight, which allows for a solid push-off from the ground. And the largest muscle in our bodies—the gluteus maximus—really only engages while we run. Numerous sweat glands and little body hair also make for a very efficient cooling system. So although we are no match for four-legged animals in a quick sprint, when it comes to covering long distances over many hours, few could keep up.

# YOUR RUNNING ROUTINE

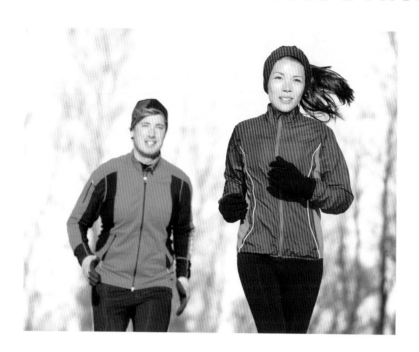

running sessions, paying close attention to your body's response. If you overdo it, running too hard or too long or too often—ease back on your running schedule until you feel yourself getting stronger.

Remember—everyone's body is unique, so don't get frustrated if you are not getting immediate results. Find your own pace.

### Too Much of a Good Thing

Running makes you feel great, and turning it into a habit can do wonders for you physically and mentally. But some runners turn that habit into an addiction, pushing themselves to run ever farther, faster, and more frequently. Not only is this bad for them psychologically—they let family, friends, work, and community take second place to the need for additional running hours or run no matter how ill or fatigued—it also places them at risk for debilitating injury. Remember: even good things taken to the extreme can be bad for you.

days. Don't worry if you get tired—alternate running and walking at a pace that feels right for your body.

During the third week, jog or run for 20 minutes, again three times on nonconsecutive days. If you need to pause, take a walking break, but don't stop. Keep yourself moving, and start running when you feel good again.

As the weeks pass, slowly increase the intensity, duration, and frequency of your

## DRESSING TO RUN

No special clothing is required for running—just be sure to wear weather-appropriate attire (and avoid running at all during extreme weather, whether hot or frigid). In warm weather, light-colored, loose-fitting clothing will help your body breathe and cool itself naturally. Synthetic fabrics, which wick away moisture, are also better than natural cotton, which holds sweat. Sunglasses and a visor are also recommended to protect your eyes from any of the sun's harmful rays. In cold weather, go for layers. Next to your skin wear synthetic or silk undergarments, such as long johns. Over that, add an insulating layer, such as fleece, and, over it all, add wind and weatherproof outer garments. A neck gaiter, bandanna, or balaclava can also protect your neck and face from the elements. And don't forget your hat—you lose much of your body heat through your head.

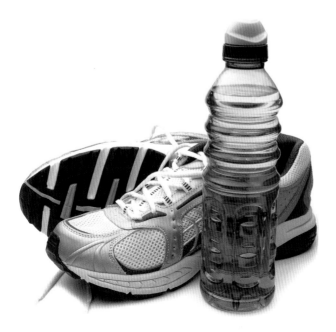

## EXERCISE EXTRAS

To aid you while performing the exercises in your running routine, take advantage of everyday objects around the house: grasp a mop handle for balance or use steps for lunges and calf exercises.

Many of the featured exercises incorporate equipment—all reasonably small tools that add variety and challenge to your workout.

**Hand weights and dumbbells.** Start with very light, 2-pound weights (or even lighter substitutes, such as unopened food cans or water bottles), and then work your way up to heavier ones. Both hand weights and dumbbells add resistance, increasing the benefits of many exercises. You can use either one for any exercise that calls for a weight. If you decide to invest in a set of dumbbells, look for an adjustable model that allows you to easily vary the weight levels. Be sure it comes with a solid-locking mechanism that makes adding and subtracting weight disks fast and easy.

**Swiss ball.** Also known as an exercise ball, fitness ball, body ball, or balance ball, this heavy-duty inflatable ball is available in a variety of sizes, with diameters ranging from 18 to 30 inches. Be sure to find the best size for your height and weight (when you sit on the ball, your thighs should be parallel or slightly above parallel to the floor). A Swiss ball is an excellent fitness aid that really works your core. Because it is unstable, you must constantly adjust your balance while performing a movement, which helps you improve your overall sense of balance and your flexibility.

**Medicine ball.** A small, weighted medicine ball, which is used like a free weight, can also be used in any exercise that calls for a hand weight.

**Resistance band.** Also known as "fitness band," "Thera-Band," "Dyna-Band," "stretching band," and "exercise band," this

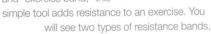

simple tool adds resistance to an exercise. You will see two types of resistance bands, one with handles and one without; both are amazing pieces of fitness equipment, which effectively tone and strengthen your entire body. Bands act in a similar way to hand weights, but unlike weights,

which rely on gravity to determine the resistance, bands use constant tension—supplied by your muscles—to add resistance to your movements and improve your overall coordination. Loop resistance bands are also available. These smaller elastics will add resistance to lower-leg and ankle exercises.

**Foam roller.** Rollers come in a variety of sizes, materials, and densities, and they can be used for stretching, strengthening, balance training, stability training, and self-massage. If you do not have access to a foam roller, you can substitute a pool noodle or a homemade towel roller. To make a towel roller, place two bath towels together, firmly roll them lengthwise, and then wrap the ends with tape. Although a towel roller works well, the dense foam of the roller will provide you with the best results.

**Aerobic step.** A portable platform with adjustable risers allows you to effectively work your calf muscles. If you don't have one, use any stable raised surface, such as a stair.

## Running Shoes

Running requires a proper pair of running shoes that support your feet and help to protect your body from injury. Choosing an appropriate pair starts with knowing your feet. You may think you know your size, but if possible have each foot measured at a reputable store that specializes in sports footwear. Determine your arch shape, which affects how you move or run. Are yours normal or high, or are you flat-footed? Also determine if you have a tendency to over- or underpronate the foot.

All of these factors will help you choose the right kind of shoe for your unique way of running, whether ones that stabilize, cushion, or control motion. Once you've found the perfect shoes, don't just lace them up and go. Take the time to break them in gradually. And don't keep running in an old pair of shoes— most last between 300 to 500 miles.

## Sports Bras

For women, a comfortable bra is essential. The right running bra will work a delicate balance between adequate support and comfort. You want to find one that minimizes movement but doesn't constrict or bind. Look for one made of a moisture-wicking fabric that is relatively seamfree to prevent chafing.

# YOUR RUNNING ROUTINE

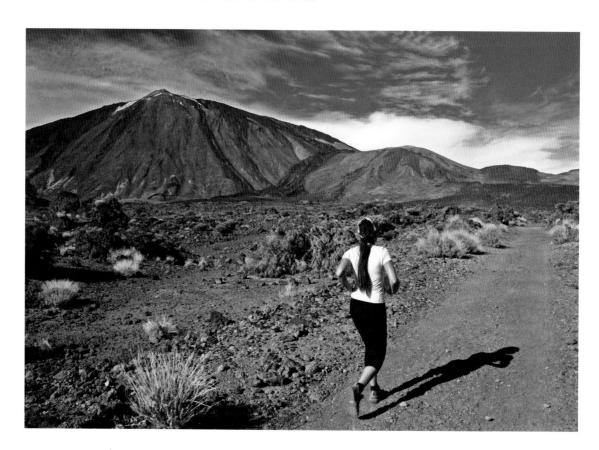

### WHERE TO RUN

You can run just about anywhere, on just about any surface, from soft sand to hard concrete, but be aware that your body will react to the impact in different ways. Changing up your running routine now and then is a smart plan—by switching between a variety of surfaces you can better strengthen muscles, ligaments, and tendons, and lower the risk of repetitive-strain injuries and muscle imbalances.

### Grass

Close-cropped grass is one of the best surfaces upon which to run. It is a soft, low-impact surface that works your muscles hard, which will build strength, and flat grass is an excellent option for speed work. Grass does have its cons, though—it is often uneven and can pose danger for runners with weak ankles. Longer grass may also hide hazards such as animal holes or rocks. Grass also turns slippery when wet, so if your regular routine takes you through grassland, plan an alternate route on rainy days.

### Woodland Trails

Many parks and forests have woodland trails that seem designed for runners, with changing scenery that makes for an interesting run. Well-maintained, level trails of soft, well-drained peat or wood chips are easy on the legs, leading to well-rounded development of your muscles, ligaments, tendons, and joints. Not all trails are equal, though—without maintenance, these surfaces can deteriorate. In forests, tree roots or other debris may present tripping hazards, and in wet weather, trails can turn muddy and slippery.

### Dirt/Earth

This category covers quite a lot of ground, from rural roads to urban parks. Depending on where you live, the composition of dirt can range from dry, sandy soil to moist, clay earth. Most dry dirt surfaces will be medium to soft, which decreases your risk of injury from excessive training. It also reduces the impact of downhill running. Wet weather, unfortunately, turns a dirt trail into slippery mud. Running in mud places added stress on vulnerable areas such as calves and Achilles tendons and increases your risk of injury.

### Synthetic Track

Outdoor tracks are ideal for speed work and interval training, with flat, forgiving surfaces and easy-to-measure distances. Yet many runners may find tracks less than exciting—it can get very boring very quickly to simply run in a circle. Running on a track may also increase your risk of injury. Those two long curves on every lap means you tend to land harder on the inside leg or pronate your foot, which can place extra stress on your ankles, knees, and hips.

### Asphalt

One of the most common road surfaces, asphalt is also one of the fastest surfaces on which to run. At its best it is a predictable, even surface that places no added stress on your Achilles tendon; at its worst, it presents traffic, potholes, and a hard, unforgiving surface. Many asphalt roads are cambered or banked on the sides, which may cause you to run with an imbalanced stride that could lead to a foot, ankle, knee, hip, or muscle injury.

### Sand

Like dirt, sand varies a great deal, from a flat, firmly packed surface to a loose, uneven one. Flat and firm is ideal, offering a forgiving, low-impact surface. Running on dunes provides good resistance training and a leg-strengthening workout. Running in soft sand will really work your calf muscles while going easy on your joints, but it does mean a higher risk of Achilles tendon injury. Running on beach sand is also a very pleasant way to pass the time, with ocean breezes and lovely scenery. Sand also gives you the opportunity to shed your shoes and run barefoot.

### Concrete

Concrete may just be a fact of life for city runners—most pavements are made up of this cement-based surface. Its accessibility is its chief charm, but it is the surface hardest on a runner's legs. Add to that the hazards of curbs, pedestrians, and stop-and-go traffic signals, and this surface is less than ideal.

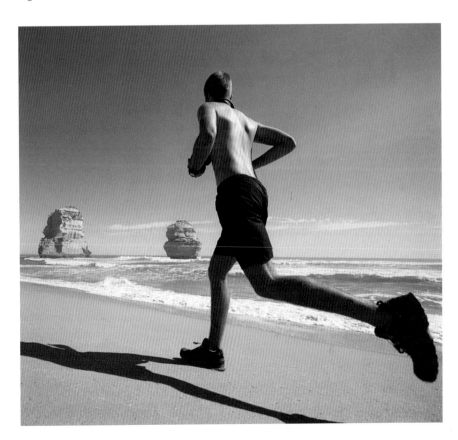

# RUNNING INJURY PRIMER

Adopting a running routine has numerous physical benefits, but your joints and muscles can take a pounding, leaving them susceptible to injury. Learning to recognize and avoid common running injuries is essential to a successful running routine.

Pushing yourself too hard, past your unique limitations, is a major cause of many running injuries. Beginners may run too often or too far, before they have become fully conditioned, and advanced runners may begin to add distance or speed, tackle rougher terrain, or run in any weather. Always keep in mind your particular body design, and adapt your expectations to account for your real strengths and weaknesses.

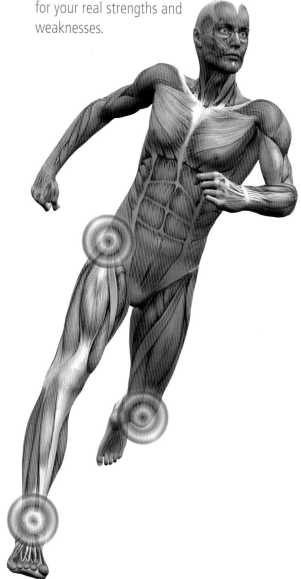

## COMMON INJURIES

Your hips, knees, legs, and feet do most of the work of running, and therefore are the body parts most vulnerable to injury. Here are some of the most common injuries runners face, their usual causes and symptoms, and the typical treatments for relieving them. Keep in mind that every individual may experience symptoms differently, but if you think you have sustained an injury, consult a physician.

### Runner's knee

A dull pain around the front of the knee (patella) where it connects with the lower end of the thigh bone (femur) is the primary symptom of runner's knee, also known as patellofemoral pain syndrome. It is commonly due to the kneecap being out of alignment. Its causes can be structural, such as a kneecap located too high in the knee joint, or induced, such as running with the feet rolling in, while the thigh muscles pull the kneecap outward.

### Causes
- Structural defects
- Weak thigh muscles
- Tight hamstrings or Achilles tendons
- Improper foot support
- Improper form
- Excessive training or overuse

### Symptoms
- Pain in and around the kneecap when going up or down stairs
- Pain in and around the kneecap when squatting

- Pain in and around the kneecap while sitting with the knee bent for a long time
- A feeling of knee weakness or instability
- Rubbing, grinding, or clicking sound when bending or straightening the knee
- Kneecap is tender to the touch

### Treatment
- Cessation of running routine until injury is healed
- Cold packs, compression, and elevation
- Pain-relief medication, such as ibuprofen
- Stretching exercises
- Strengthening exercises
- Adding arch support in shoes

## Shin splint

Pain running along the front or inside of the shin bone (tibia) is a common runner's complaint. Many runners incur shin splints when they boost their running routine too quickly—adding too many miles or running too often without giving the body a chance to properly recover from strenuous activity. Like runner's knee the causes may be structural or induced. Shin splints involve damage to one of two groups of muscles along the shin bone. An anterolateral shin splint affects the front and outer part of the shin muscles and is caused by a structural imbalance in the size of opposite muscles. A posteromedial shin splint affects the back and inner part of the muscles of the shin. Any running can cause a posteromedial shin splint, as well as running in improper shoes. People with flat feet are also prone to shin splints.

### Causes
- Structural defects
- Improper foot support
- Improper form
- Excessive training or overuse

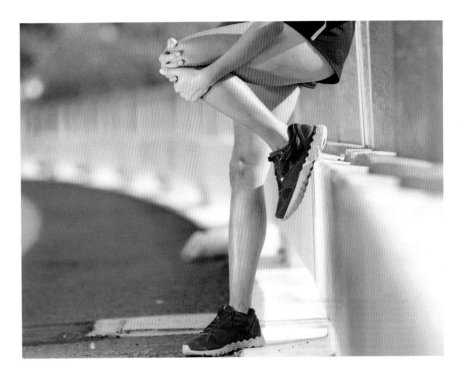

### Symptoms
- Pain on the front and outside of the shin when the heel touches the ground while running that eventually becomes constant (anterolateral)
- Pain on the inside of the lower leg above the ankle that eventually becomes constant (posteromedial).
- Shin is painful to the touch (posteromedial)
- Pain when standing on the toes or rolling the ankle inward (posteromedial)
- Inflammation (posteromedial)

### Treatment
- Cessation of running routine until injury is healed
- Stretching exercises
- Strengthening exercises
- Cold packs
- Pain-relief medication, such as ibuprofen
- Wearing running shoes with a rigid heel
- Adding arch support in shoes
- Slow return to activity after several weeks of healing

# RUNNING INJURY PRIMER

### Plantar fasciitis

Plantar fasciitis is an inflammation of the thick band of tissue in the bottom of the foot that extends from the heel to the toes, called the plantar fascia. Plantar fasciitis produces severe pain in the heel, especially when you stand up after resting. If you are overweight, work in an occupation that requires a lot of walking or standing on hard surfaces, have flat feet, or have high arches, you may be susceptible to plantar fasciitis and should keep this in mind as you develop your running routine.

**Causes**
- Excessive training or overuse
- Tight calf muscles

**Symptoms**
- Severe pain in the heel of the foot

**Treatment**
- Rest
- Cold packs
- Nonsteroidal anti-inflammatory medications
- Stretching exercises

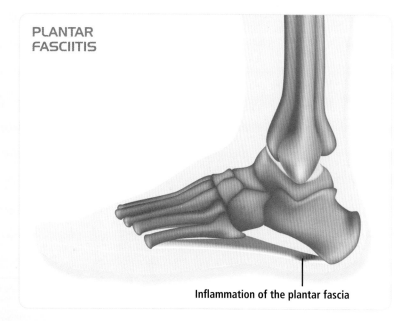

PLANTAR
FASCIITIS

**Inflammation of the plantar fascia**

### Ankle sprain

An ankle sprain is the stretching or tearing of the ankle ligaments (the tough bands of elastic tissue that connect bones to one another). You are most likely to incur a sprain when your foot twists or rolls inward. The symptom and treatment of ankle sprains vary depending on the severity of the stretching or tearing.

**Causes**
- Awkward foot placement
- Running or walking on irregular surfaces
- Weak muscles
- Loose ligaments
- Improper footwear

**Symptoms**
- Swelling
- Pain
- Bruising

**Treatment**
- Resting the ankle
- Wrapping the ankle with elastic bandage or tape
- Cold packs
- Elevating the ankle
- Gradual return to walking and exercise
- A walking cast (for moderate sprains)
- Surgery (for severe sprains)
- Physical therapy (for severe sprains)

### Stress fractures

Most often occurring in the lower leg or the foot, stress fractures are tiny fissures in the surface of a bone. You are most likely to suffer from a stress fracture if you increase the intensity or frequency of your runs over several weeks or months or if your body is low in calcium. The tibia (the inner and larger bone of the leg below the knee), the femur (thigh bone), the sacrum (the triangular bone at the base of the spine), and the metatarsal (toe) bones are the most susceptible to stress fractures. If you suspect that you have one, stop your running routine, and consult a physician as soon as possible—left untreated these tiny cracks can spread to become a full bone fracture.

### Causes
- Excessive training or overuse
- Structural defects

### Symptoms
- Muscle soreness that comes on gradually in the affected area
- Stiffness in the affected area
- Pinpoint pain on the affected bone

### Treatment
- Cessation of running routine until injury is healed
- Rest
- Nonsteroidal anti-inflammatory medications
- Stretching exercises
- Muscle strengthening
- A cast or other form of immobilization of the area, depending on the severity of the injury
- Physical therapy (for severe fractures)

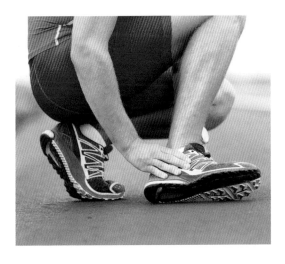

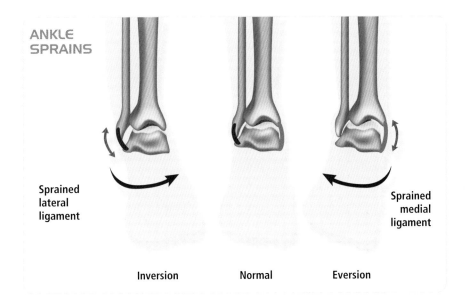

ANKLE SPRAINS

Sprained lateral ligament

Sprained medial ligament

Inversion    Normal    Eversion

## Iliotibial band syndrome

Iliotibial band syndrome, usually shortened to IT band syndrome or simply ITBS, affects the long ligament that runs along the outside of the thigh, from the top of the hip to the outside of the knee. ITBS occurs when this ligament thickens and rubs the knee bone, producing inflammation. Certain structural factors may make you more susceptible, such as a difference in length between one leg and the other. How you run and where you run also plays a role in the development of ITBS; for example, long-distance runners are more likely to develop ITBS.

### Causes
- Tight or wide iliotibial band
- Weak hip muscles
- Overpronation of the feet
- Excessive training or overuse
- Excessive hill running
- Running on cambered surfaces
- Difference in leg length

### Symptoms
- Pain occurring on the outside of the knee
- Tightness in the iliotibial band

# RUNNING INJURY PRIMER

- Pain aggravated by running, particularly downhill
- Pain during flexion or extension of the knee
- Weakness in hip abduction

### Treatment
- Rest
- Avoiding painful stimuli, such as downhill running
- Cold packs after you run
- Decreasing the frequency, duration, or intensity of your runs
- Heat and stretching prior to exercise
- Self-massage

### Blisters

These fluid-filled bubbles on the surface of the skin can ruin anyone's run. Not only are blisters painful, they can also alter your gait, which may lead to more serious injuries of the leg and hip. To reduce any friction between your feet and socks/shoes, wear well-fitted shoes and seamless, moisture-wicking socks. Try spreading petroleum jelly on blister-prone areas, too.

## Muscle strain

Some of the most common injuries runners suffer are muscle strains, also called muscle pulls. These are small tears in a muscle, caused by stretching the fibers beyond capacity. The hamstrings, quadriceps, calf muscles, and groin muscles are the most frequent sites of strains. A popping sensation in the affected area is a typical sign that you have strained a muscle.

### Causes
- Overstretching a muscle
- Excessive training or overuse
- Fatigue
- Falling

### Symptoms
- A sudden, sharp pain in the affected area
- Muscle stiffness, soreness, and tightness
- Swelling or bruising (moderate and severe strains)

### Treatment
- Rest
- Cold packs
- Compression
- Elevation of affected area

## Achilles tendonitis

Runners often experience the effects of Achilles tendonitis. The Achilles tendon, running from the heel to lower calf, is the largest and most vulnerable tendon in the body and joins the gastrocnemius (calf) and the soleus muscles of the lower leg to the heel of the foot. Although the Achilles tendon is strong, it is not very flexible—stretching it beyond its capacity can result in inflammation, ruptures, and tears. Although Achilles tendonitis is a chronic injury, its symptoms can come on suddenly or appear if a bout of acute tendonitis fails to heal properly. If you suspect that you may have developed this injury, don't try to push through the pain; instead stop and rest immediately.

### Causes
- Lack of flexibility in the calf muscles
- Excessive training or overuse

### Symptoms
- Pain in the back of the ankle and just above the heel
- Pain that increases during running

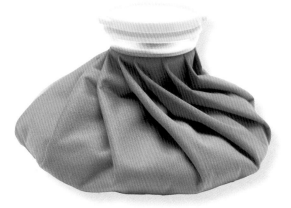

## MUSCLE ACTIVATION AND THE GAIT CYCLE

Running may be a natural human activity, but to derive the most benefit from running, proper form is essential. The first step is to understand the gait cycle, or the rhythmic alternating movements of the legs and feet that result in the forward movement of the body—in other words, how you run. A gait cycle begins when one foot makes contact with the ground and ends when that same foot makes contact with the ground again. It consists of two phases: the stance (or support) phase and the swing (or unsupported) phase. A running gait consists of the following:

**Stance phase.** Begins when the heel of the forward leg makes contact with the ground and ends when the toe of the same leg leaves the ground. This phase has three subphases.
- *Heel strike.* The heel of the forward foot touches the ground.
- *Midstance.* The foot is flat on the ground, and the weight of the body is directly over the supporting limb. In midstance, as your other foot is in swing phase, all your body weight is borne by a single leg, which means that your lower leg is particularly susceptible to injury.

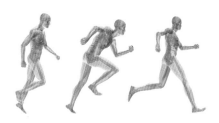

- *Toe-off.* Only the big toe of the forward foot is in contact with the ground. During toe-off, your foot should be supinated (rotated outward), allowing the bones of the midfoot to brace against each other, which forms a rigid structure that propels the body weight forward. Improper running shoes or an abnormally pronating foot can prevent the correct functioning of the foot in this phase, increasing the risk of injury.

The quadriceps and rectus femoris work as knee extensors, while the rectus femoris also contributes to hip flexion. These muscles engage in anticipation of and during the stance phase to support the body. The rectus femoris also activates in mid-swing phase, working as a hip flexor.

**Swing phase.** Begins when the foot is no longer in contact with the ground. The leg is free to move. This phase has two subphases.
- *Acceleration.* The swinging limb catches up to and passes the torso.
- *Deceleration.* Forward movement of the limb is slowed down to position the foot for heel strike.

Most muscles work in pairs, with an antagonist muscle working in opposition to an agonist. The major antagonist muscles to the quadriceps are the gluteal muscles, which extend the hip, and the hamstrings, which extend the hip and flex the knee. The hamstring muscles activate in mid-swing phase to help decelerate the lower leg. In late swing phase and in the first half of the stance phase, both groups engage to begin extending the hip.

Lower-leg muscles acting on the ankle are the tibialis anterior, gastrocnemius, and soleus. The gastrocnemius and soleus are active in the last part of swing phase to prepare for foot strike and remain active through the stance phase until just before toe-off in order to propel the body forward.

---

- Pain that eases as you warm up and stretch the tendon
- Pinpoint tenderness or soreness that increases when palpated
- Small lumps and bumps over the area of the tendon

### Treatment
- Reducing your running routine
- Avoiding speed training and hill running
- Pre-run stretching exercises that target the Achilles tendon
- Post-run cold packs

## Lower-back pain
Running often places a high level of stress on the lower back, and the repetitive motion may aggravate existing lumbar problems or even bring on persistent or intermittent lower-back pain.

### Causes
- Tight or weak lower-back muscles

### Symptoms
- Pain and stiffness in the lumbar spine area
- Pain or a tingling sensation running from the lower back through the leg

### Treatment
- Warming up before running
- Stretching exercises
- Strengthening exercises
- Wearing properly fitted running-specific shoes
- Running on forgiving surfaces
- Cold packs

# FULL-BODY ANATOMY

ANNOTATION KEY
* indicates deep muscles

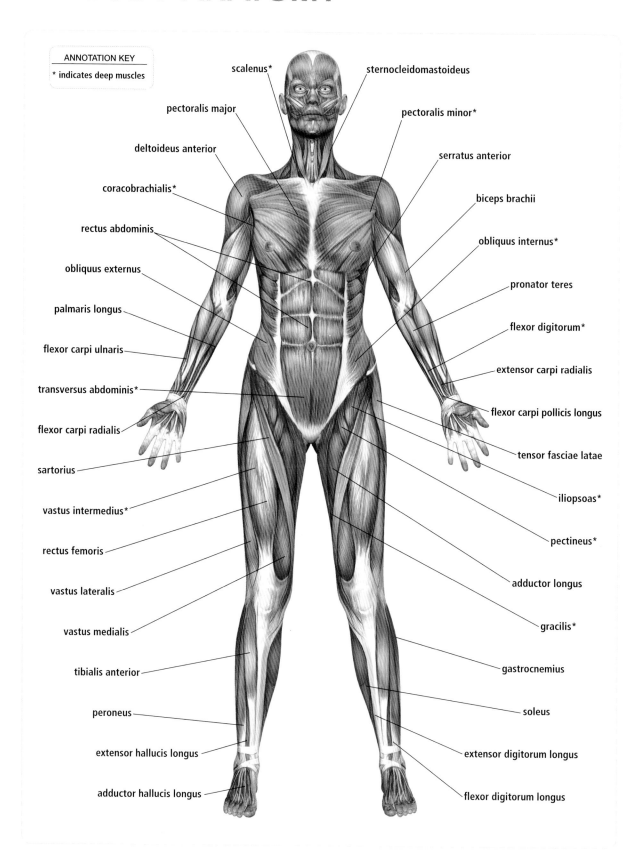

scalenus*

sternocleidomastoideus

pectoralis major

pectoralis minor*

deltoideus anterior

serratus anterior

coracobrachialis*

biceps brachii

rectus abdominis

obliquus internus*

obliquus externus

pronator teres

palmaris longus

flexor digitorum*

flexor carpi ulnaris

extensor carpi radialis

transversus abdominis*

flexor carpi pollicis longus

flexor carpi radialis

tensor fasciae latae

sartorius

iliopsoas*

vastus intermedius*

pectineus*

rectus femoris

adductor longus

vastus lateralis

gracilis*

vastus medialis

gastrocnemius

tibialis anterior

soleus

peroneus

extensor hallucis longus

extensor digitorum longus

adductor hallucis longus

flexor digitorum longus

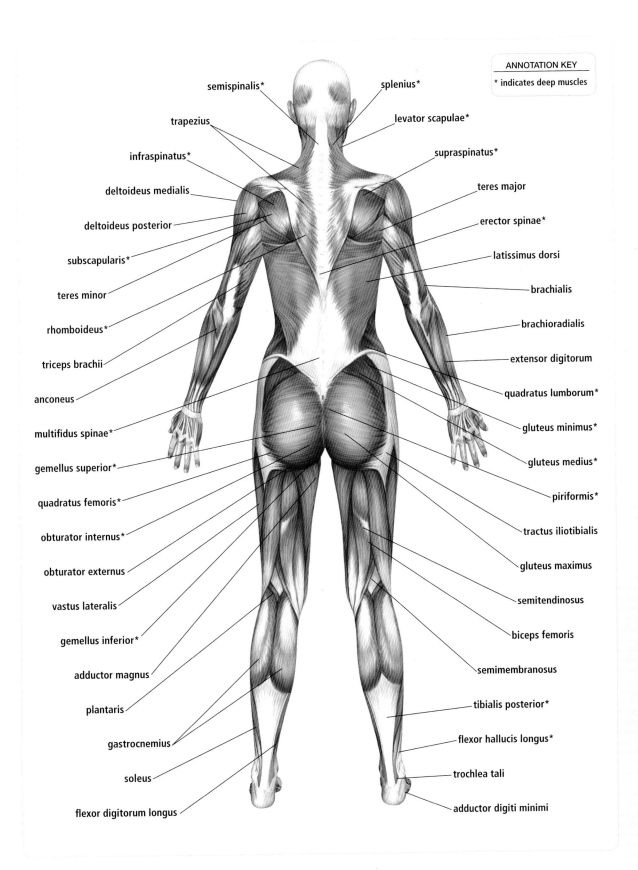

semispinalis*

splenius*

trapezius

levator scapulae*

infraspinatus*

supraspinatus*

deltoideus medialis

teres major

deltoideus posterior

erector spinae*

subscapularis*

latissimus dorsi

teres minor

brachialis

rhomboideus*

brachioradialis

triceps brachii

extensor digitorum

anconeus

quadratus lumborum*

multifidus spinae*

gluteus minimus*

gemellus superior*

gluteus medius*

quadratus femoris*

piriformis*

obturator internus*

tractus iliotibialis

obturator externus

gluteus maximus

vastus lateralis

semitendinosus

gemellus inferior*

biceps femoris

adductor magnus

semimembranosus

plantaris

tibialis posterior*

gastrocnemius

flexor hallucis longus*

soleus

trochlea tali

flexor digitorum longus

adductor digiti minimi

ANNOTATION KEY

* indicates deep muscles

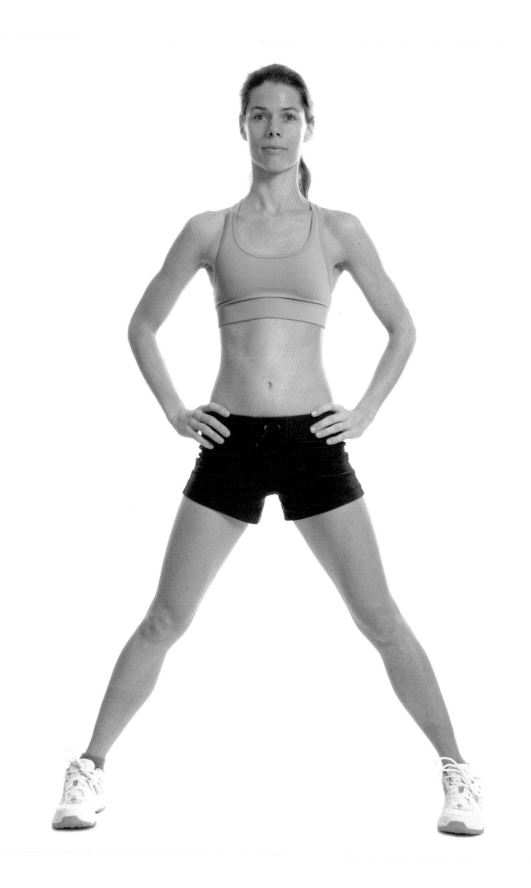

# RUNNERS' STRETCHES

As with any kind of exercise, before setting off on a run, it is important to warm up and stretch your muscles. Stretching exercises lengthen the muscle fibers, increasing their functionality. With regular pre-run and post-run stretching, you will see not only greater flexibility but also improved posture, balance, and range of motion. The following pages feature stretches that focus on the primary running muscles—the quadriceps, hamstrings, glutes, calves, ankles, and hip flexors, as well as secondary areas such as the lumbar spine. Do a fast 5-to-10-minute cardiovascular warm-up, and then perform a series of these before a run. After a run, a few of these stretches will form a perfect cool-down regimen.

# STANDING QUADRICEPS STRETCH

**1** Stand with your feet together. Bend your left leg behind you, and grasp your foot with your left hand. Pull your heel toward your buttocks until you feel a stretch in the front of your thigh. Keep both knees together and aligned.

**2** Hold for 15 seconds. Repeat sequence three times on each leg.

## BEST FOR

- **rectus femoris**
- **vastus lateralis**
- **vastus medialis**
- **vastus intermedius**

**TARGETS**
- Quadriceps

**LEVEL**
- Beginner

**BENEFITS**
- Helps to keep thigh muscles flexible

**NOT ADVISABLE IF YOU HAVE . . .**
- Knee issues

**MODIFICATION**
**Easier:** Wrap a resistance band or small towel around your ankle and grasp both ends to aid in raising your foot.

**AVOID**
- Leaning forward with your chest.
- Bringing your foot closer to your buttocks than you can reach with a comfortable stretch—this can compress the knee joint.

**DO IT RIGHT**
- Both knees to remain pressed together.
- With the arm opposite your bent leg, lean against a wall or other stable object to aid your balance.

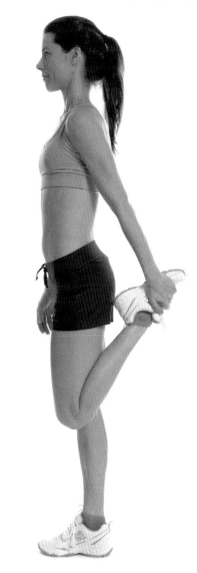

tensor fasciae latae

vastus intermedius*

rectus femoris

vastus lateralis

vastus medialis

**ANNOTATION KEY**

**Black text indicates target muscles**

Gray text indicates other working muscles

\* indicates deep muscles

# SPRINTER STRETCH

1. Kneel with your left knee bent, your toe pointed and extended behind you on the floor. Bend your right leg so that your right foot is flat on the floor, next to your left knee.

2. Position your hands on the floor just beyond shoulder-width apart, slightly in front of your body, with palms downward.

3. Sit back on your left heel as you lean slightly forward.

4. Release the stretch, switch legs, and repeat.

**AVOID**
- Allowing your foot to roll inward.

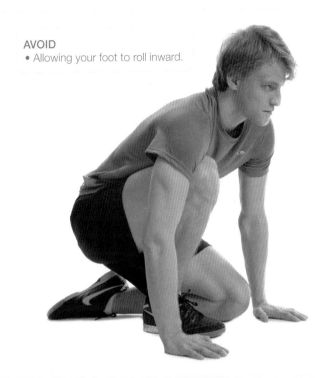

**DO IT RIGHT**
- Keep the sole of your front foot and the upper arch of your back foot on the floor.
- Lean your chest farther forward over your raised upper leg to increase the intensity of the stretch.

**BEST FOR**

- soleus
- extensor digitorum longus
- tendo calcaneus

**TARGETS**
- Achilles tendon
- Calves

**LEVEL**
- Beginner

**BENEFITS**
- Strengthens and stretches the Achilles tendon
- Stretches calf muscles

**NOT ADVISABLE IF YOU HAVE . . .**
- Knee issues

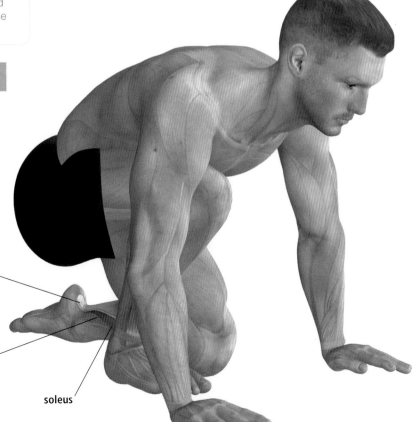

*tendo calcaneus*

extensor digitorum longus

soleus

**ANNOTATION KEY**
Black text indicates target muscles
*Black italics indicates tendons*

# FORWARD LUNGE

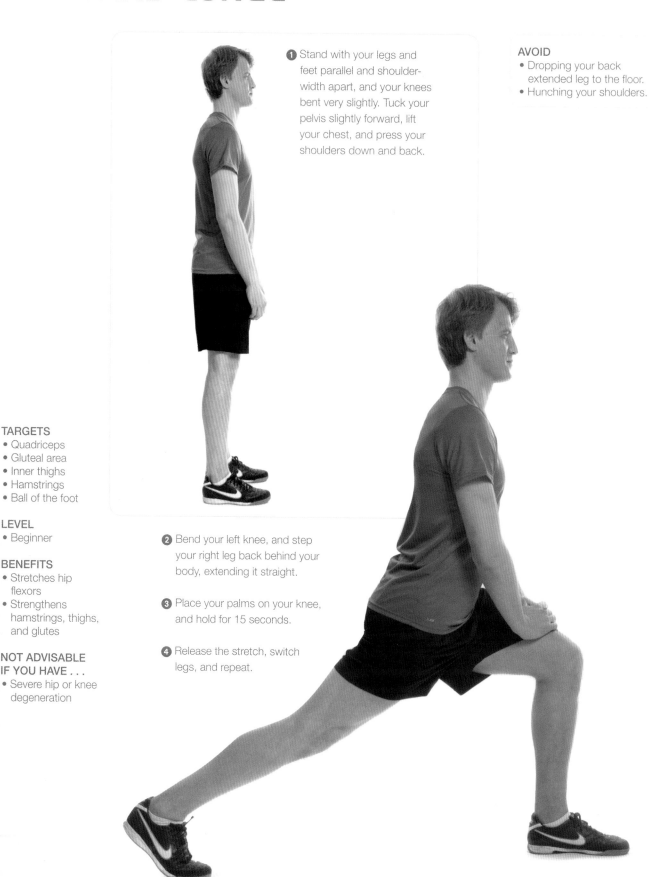

**①** Stand with your legs and feet parallel and shoulder-width apart, and your knees bent very slightly. Tuck your pelvis slightly forward, lift your chest, and press your shoulders down and back.

**AVOID**
- Dropping your back extended leg to the floor.
- Hunching your shoulders.

**TARGETS**
- Quadriceps
- Gluteal area
- Inner thighs
- Hamstrings
- Ball of the foot

**LEVEL**
- Beginner

**BENEFITS**
- Stretches hip flexors
- Strengthens hamstrings, thighs, and glutes

**NOT ADVISABLE IF YOU HAVE . . .**
- Severe hip or knee degeneration

**②** Bend your left knee, and step your right leg back behind your body, extending it straight.

**③** Place your palms on your knee, and hold for 15 seconds.

**④** Release the stretch, switch legs, and repeat.

**DO IT RIGHT**
- Keep your back leg extended in line with your hips to form one long straight line.
- Keep your knee directly above your ankle.

**BEST FOR**
- rectus femoris
- vastus lateralis
- vastus intermedius
- vastus medialis
- biceps femoris
- semitendinosus
- semimembranosus
- gluteus maximus
- adductor longus
- adductor magnus
- adductor brevis
- iliopsoas
- gracilis
- pectineus
- tensor fasciae latae
- obturator externus
- gluteus minimus

**ANNOTATION KEY**

Black text indicates target muscles

* indicates deep muscles

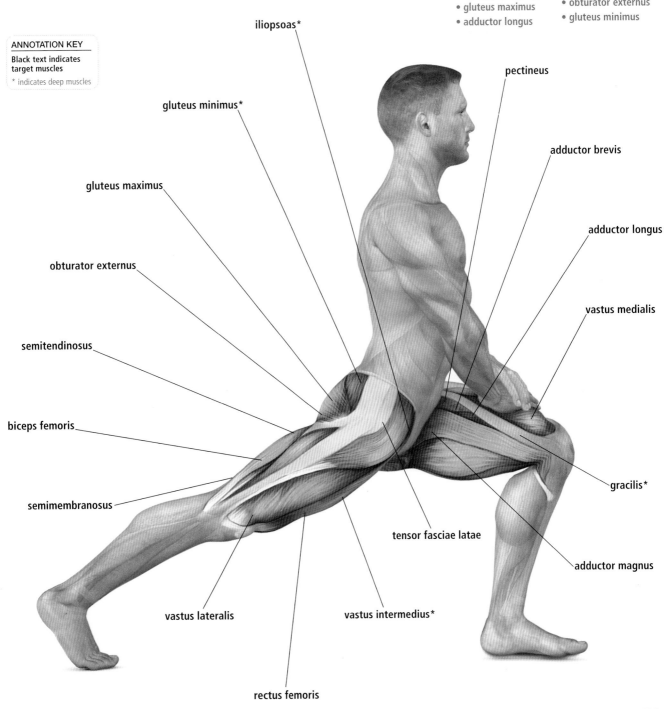

iliopsoas*

gluteus minimus*

gluteus maximus

obturator externus

semitendinosus

biceps femoris

semimembranosus

vastus lateralis

rectus femoris

vastus intermedius*

tensor fasciae latae

pectineus

adductor brevis

adductor longus

vastus medialis

gracilis*

adductor magnus

# FORWARD LUNGE WITH TWIST

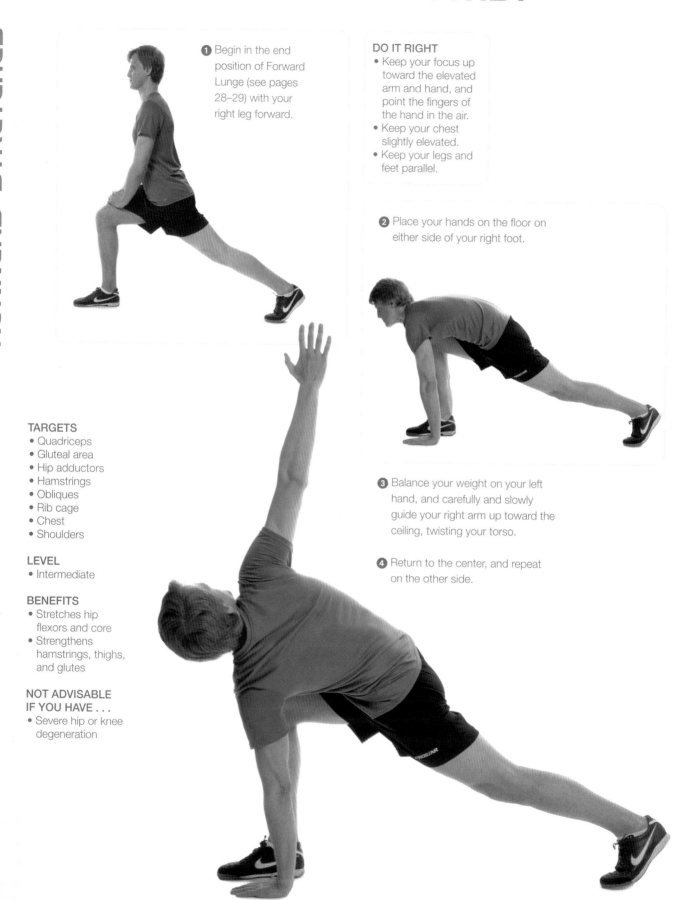

**1** Begin in the end position of Forward Lunge (see pages 28–29) with your right leg forward.

**DO IT RIGHT**
- Keep your focus up toward the elevated arm and hand, and point the fingers of the hand in the air.
- Keep your chest slightly elevated.
- Keep your legs and feet parallel.

**2** Place your hands on the floor on either side of your right foot.

**3** Balance your weight on your left hand, and carefully and slowly guide your right arm up toward the ceiling, twisting your torso.

**4** Return to the center, and repeat on the other side.

**TARGETS**
- Quadriceps
- Gluteal area
- Hip adductors
- Hamstrings
- Obliques
- Rib cage
- Chest
- Shoulders

**LEVEL**
- Intermediate

**BENEFITS**
- Stretches hip flexors and core
- Strengthens hamstrings, thighs, and glutes

**NOT ADVISABLE IF YOU HAVE . . .**
- Severe hip or knee degeneration

## AVOID
- Holding your breath.
- Dropping the elevated arm behind you—look for both arms to remain on the same plane.

## BEST FOR
- rectus femoris
- vastus lateralis
- vastus intermedius
- vastus medialis
- biceps femoris
- semitendinosus
- semimembranosus
- gluteus minimus
- gluteus maximus
- obliquus externus
- obliquus internus
- adductor longus
- adductor magnus
- adductor brevis
- gracilis
- pectineus
- obturator externus
- iliopsoas
- tensor fasciae latae

## ANNOTATION KEY
Black text indicates target muscles

Gray text indicates other working muscles

* indicates deep muscles

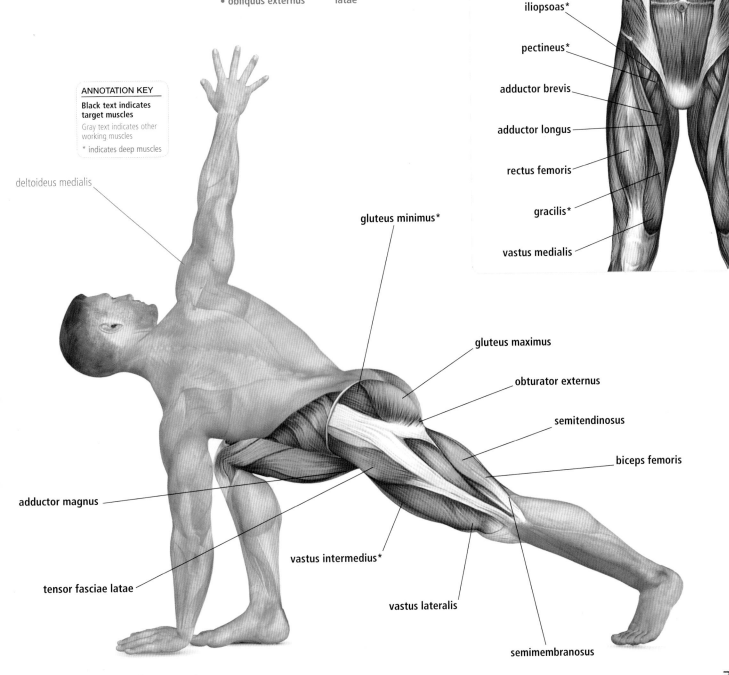

pectoralis minor*

pectoralis major

obliquus internus*

obliquus externus

iliopsoas*

pectineus*

adductor brevis

adductor longus

rectus femoris

gracilis*

vastus medialis

deltoideus medialis

gluteus minimus*

gluteus maximus

obturator externus

semitendinosus

biceps femoris

adductor magnus

vastus intermedius*

tensor fasciae latae

vastus lateralis

semimembranosus

# STRAIGHT-LEG LUNGE

**①** Stand with your legs and feet parallel and shoulder-width apart. Bend your knees very slightly and tuck your pelvis slightly forward, lift your chest, and press your shoulders downward and back.

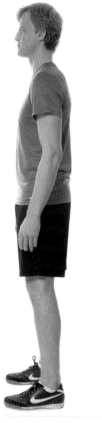

**DO IT RIGHT**
- Flex the front foot by lifting the ball of the foot off the floor to maximize the intensity of the stretch.
- Keep the heel of your back leg on the floor throughout the stretch.

**AVOID**
- Holding unnecessary tension in the upper body—relax and breathe in and out naturally.

**TARGETS**
- Hamstrings
- Lower back
- Calves

**LEVEL**
- Beginner

**BENEFITS**
- Stretches hamstrings, calves, and lower back

**NOT ADVISABLE IF YOU HAVE . . .**
- Lower-back pain

**②** Take one step forward with the right foot.

**③** Keeping your legs straight, lean your torso forward as far as possible over your right leg. Allow the weight of the upper body to intensify the stretch.

**④** Return to standing, and repeat on the other side.

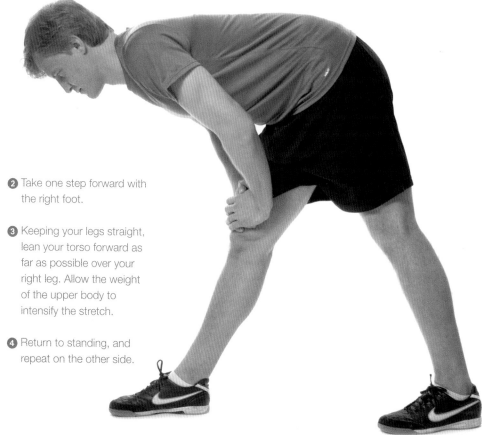

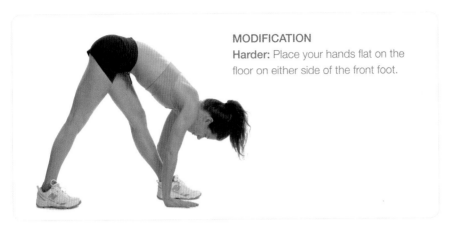

**MODIFICATION**

**Harder:** Place your hands flat on the floor on either side of the front foot.

**BEST FOR**

- biceps femoris
- semitendinosus
- semimembranosus
- erector spinae
- gastrocnemius
- soleus

**ANNOTATION KEY**

**Black text indicates target muscles**

* indicates deep muscles

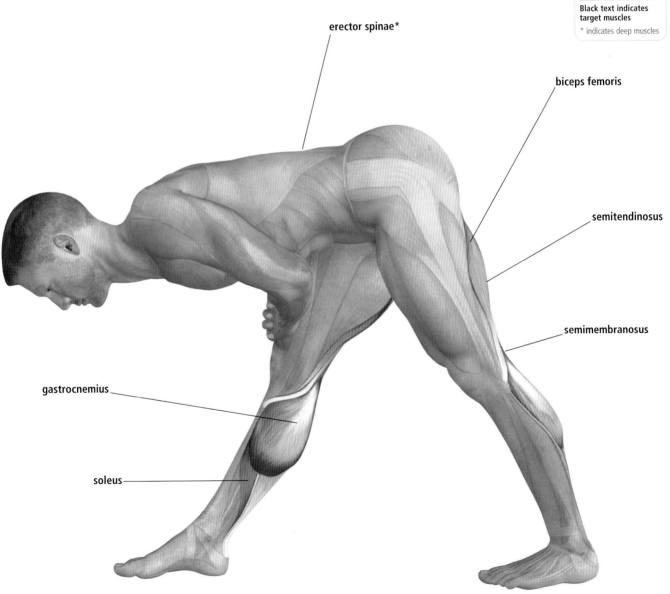

erector spinae*

biceps femoris

semitendinosus

semimembranosus

gastrocnemius

soleus

# WIDE-LEGGED FORWARD BEND

**1** Stand with your legs and feet parallel and generously outside of shoulder width. Bend your knees very slightly and tuck your pelvis slightly forward, lift your chest, and press your shoulders downward and back.

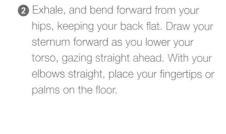

### DO IT RIGHT
- Contract your leg muscles, and keep your feet firmly grounded throughout the stretch.
- Exhale as you hinge forward from the hips.
- Keep your chest elevated.

### AVOID
- Bending forward from your waist.
- Compressing the back of your neck as you look forward.
- Tensing your shoulders.

### TARGETS
- Hamstrings
- Lower back
- Gluteal area
- Calves

### LEVEL
- Beginner

### BENEFITS
- Stretches and strengthens hamstrings, groins, and spine

### NOT ADVISABLE IF YOU HAVE . . .
- Lower-back issues

**2** Exhale, and bend forward from your hips, keeping your back flat. Draw your sternum forward as you lower your torso, gazing straight ahead. With your elbows straight, place your fingertips or palms on the floor.

**3** With another exhalation, place your hands on the floor in between your feet, and lower your torso into a full forward bend. Lengthen your spine by pulling your sit bones up toward the ceiling and drawing your head to the floor. If possible, bend your elbows and place your forehead on the floor.

**4** Hold for 30 seconds to 1 minute. To return to your starting position, straighten your elbows and raise your torso while keeping your back flat.

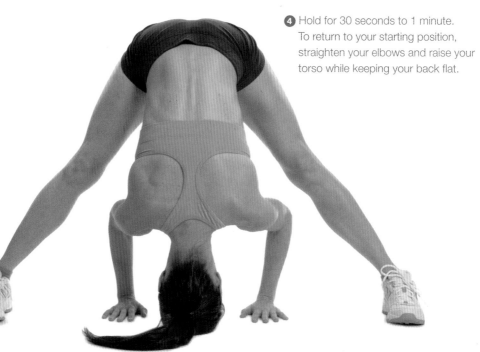

## MODIFICATION

**Easier:** Follow step 1, and then exhale, bending forward until your torso is nearly parallel to the floor. Place your hands on the floor in line with your shoulders, making sure that your lower back is straight. Hold for 15 to 30 seconds.

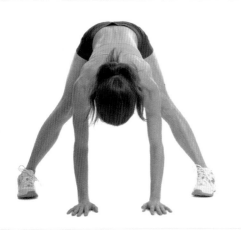

## MODIFICATION

**Easier:** Widen your stance or place a block, book, or other solid object on the floor for support.

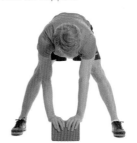

### BEST FOR

- biceps femoris
- semitendinosus
- semimembranosus
- gluteus maximus
- gluteus medius
- gluteus minimus
- rectus abdominis
- transversus abdominis
- obliquus externus
- obliquus internus
- erector spinae
- gastrocnemius
- soleus

### ANNOTATION KEY

**Black text indicates target muscles**

Gray text indicates other working muscles

\* indicates deep muscles

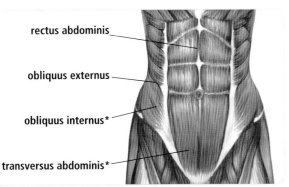

rectus abdominis

obliquus externus

obliquus internus\*

transversus abdominis\*

gluteus minimus\*

adductor magnus

quadratus femoris\*

semitendinosus

biceps femoris

semimembranosus

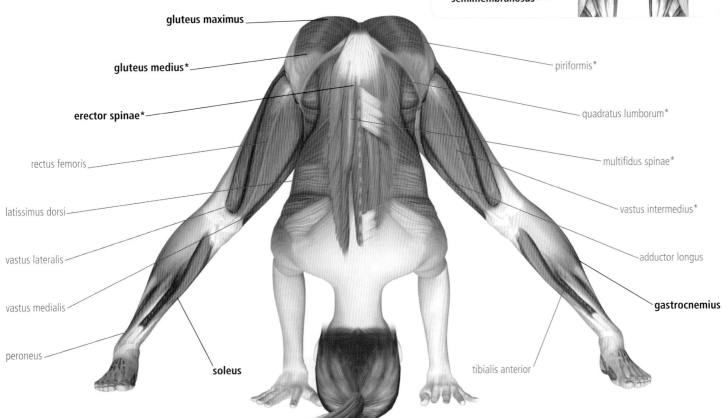

gluteus maximus

gluteus medius\*

erector spinae\*

rectus femoris

latissimus dorsi

vastus lateralis

vastus medialis

peroneus

soleus

piriformis\*

quadratus lumborum\*

multifidus spinae\*

vastus intermedius\*

adductor longus

gastrocnemius

tibialis anterior

# UNILATERAL SEATED FORWARD BEND

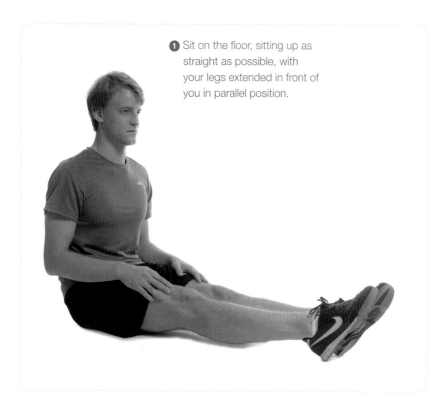

① Sit on the floor, sitting up as straight as possible, with your legs extended in front of you in parallel position.

**DO IT RIGHT**
• Drop your head to benefit your rhomboids, and for a more intense overall stretch.

**AVOID**
• Allowing the foot of your bent leg to shift beneath your straight leg.
• Straining your back—if yours is tight, try performing this stretch with a support, such as a sofa, behind you. Be sure to position your lower back as close to the support as possible.

**TARGETS**
• Hamstrings

**LEVEL**
• Beginner

**BENEFITS**
• Stretches hamstrings, groins, and spine

**NOT ADVISABLE IF YOU HAVE . . .**
• Knee injury
• Lower-back injury

② Bend your right leg until it is turned out, with the bottom of your right foot resting at your left inner thigh just above the kneecap. Rest your hands on your knee.

③ Bend from your waist, and lean forward over your left leg. Place your forearms above your left kneecap.

④ Switch legs, and repeat on the other side.

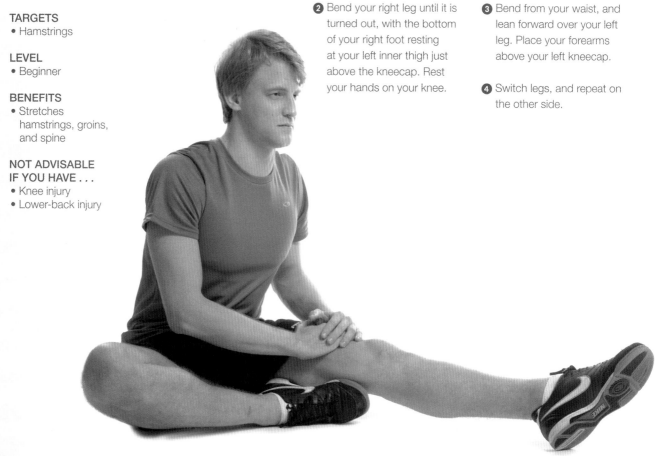

## MODIFICATION

**Harder:** Follow steps 1 through 3, then exhale and stretch your sternum forward as you fold your torso over your left leg. Grasp the inside of your left foot with your right hand. Use your left hand to guide your torso to the left.

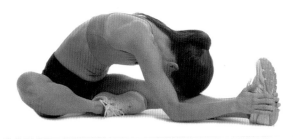

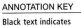

**ANNOTATION KEY**

**Black text indicates target muscles**

* indicates deep muscles

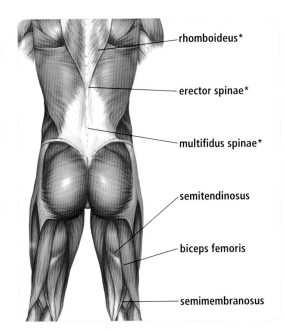

rhomboideus*

erector spinae*

multifidus spinae*

semitendinosus

biceps femoris

semimembranosus

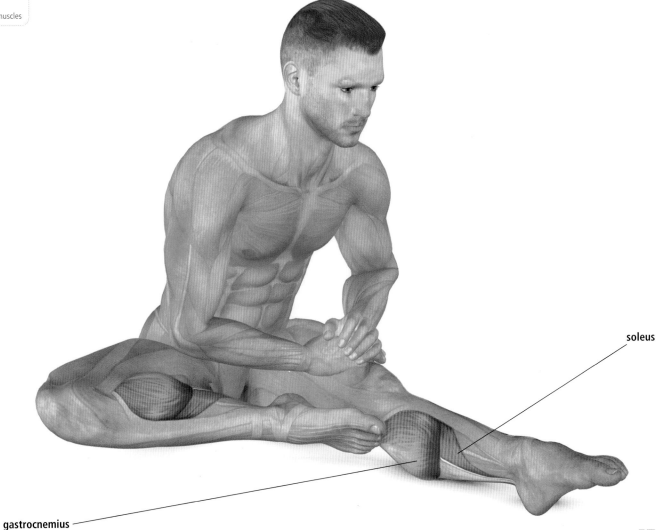

soleus

gastrocnemius

# BILATERAL SEATED FORWARD BEND

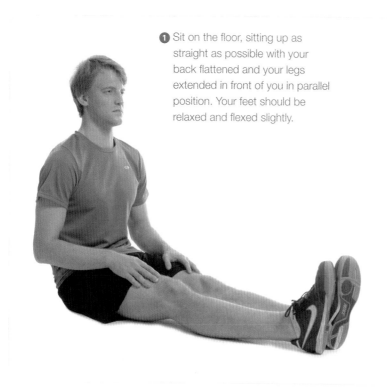

**❶** Sit on the floor, sitting up as straight as possible with your back flattened and your legs extended in front of you in parallel position. Your feet should be relaxed and flexed slightly.

### DO IT RIGHT
- Bend at the hips and keep your spine straight as you stretch.
- Extend your torso as far forward over your legs as possible.

### AVOID
- Holding your breath.
- Tensing your jaw or clenching your teeth while performing any stretch: relaxing your mouth will help you breathe evenly.

### TARGETS
- Hamstrings

### LEVEL
- Beginner

### BENEFITS
- Stretches hamstrings, groins, and spine

### NOT ADVISABLE IF YOU HAVE . . .
- Knee injury
- Lower-back injury

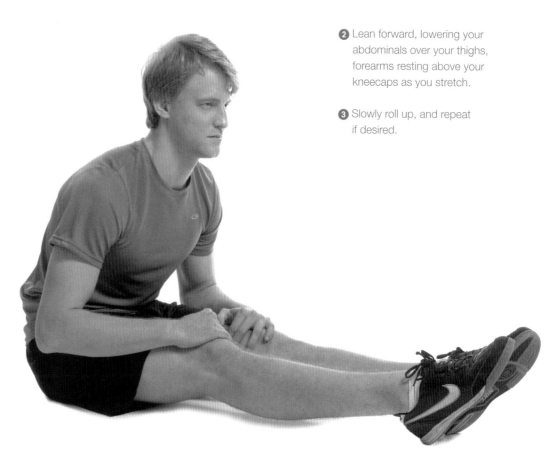

**❷** Lean forward, lowering your abdominals over your thighs, forearms resting above your kneecaps as you stretch.

**❸** Slowly roll up, and repeat if desired.

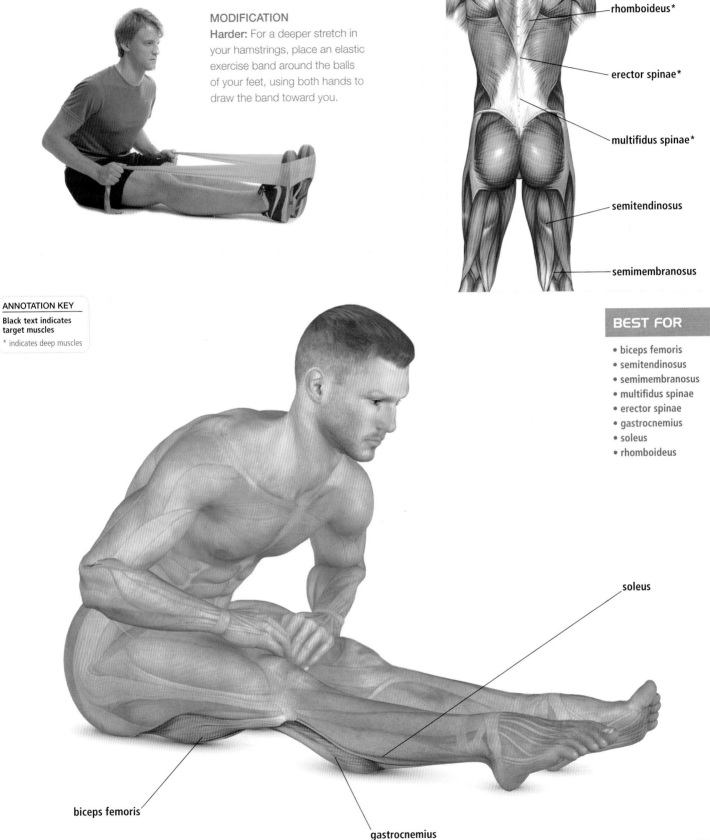

**MODIFICATION**

**Harder:** For a deeper stretch in your hamstrings, place an elastic exercise band around the balls of your feet, using both hands to draw the band toward you.

rhomboideus*

erector spinae*

multifidus spinae*

semitendinosus

semimembranosus

**ANNOTATION KEY**

**Black text indicates target muscles**

* indicates deep muscles

**BEST FOR**

- biceps femoris
- semitendinosus
- semimembranosus
- multifidus spinae
- erector spinae
- gastrocnemius
- soleus
- rhomboideus

soleus

biceps femoris

gastrocnemius

# KNEE-TO-CHEST HUG

**1** Lie supine on a mat with your legs together and arms outstretched.

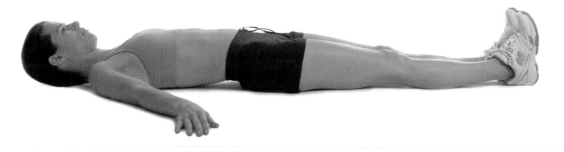

**2** Bend your right knee, and bring your foot to your body's midline while clasping your hands together to hold your knee. Hold the stretch for 15 seconds.

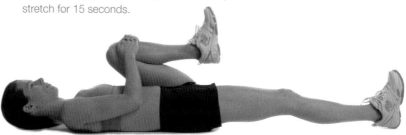

**TARGETS**
• Lower back
• Hips

**LEVEL**
• Beginner

**BENEFITS**
• Stretches lower back, hip extensors, and hip rotators

**NOT ADVISABLE IF YOU HAVE . . .**
• Advanced degenerative joint disease

**3** Return to the starting position.

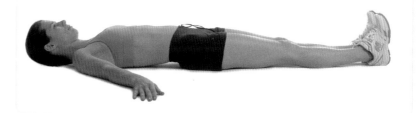

**4** Again, clasping your hands together to hold your knee, bend your right knee, but this time rotate the right leg to the left, bringing the side of your leg against your chest.

**5** Hold the stretch for 15 seconds, and then return to the starting position. Repeat the entire sequence with the left leg bent.

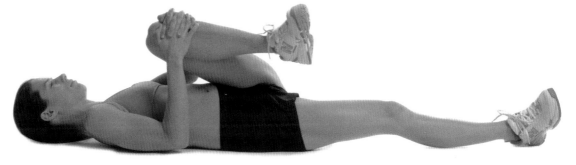

## MODIFICATION

**Similar level of difficulty:** Follow step 1, and then draw both legs to your chest.

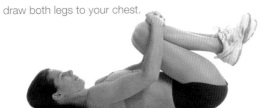

## AVOID

• Lifting your buttocks off the floor.

## DO IT RIGHT

• Keep your spine in neutral position.

### BEST FOR

- erector spinae
- latissimus dorsi
- gluteus maximus
- gluteus minimus
- piriformis
- gemellus superior
- gemellus inferior
- obturator externus
- obturator internus
- quadratus femoris

erector spinae*

piriformis*

gemellus superior*

obturator internus*

quadratus femoris*

obturator externus

gemellus inferior*

### ANNOTATION KEY

**Black text indicates target muscles**

Gray text indicates other working muscles

* indicates deep muscles

obliquus externus

latissimus dorsi

biceps femoris

gluteus minimus*

gluteus maximus

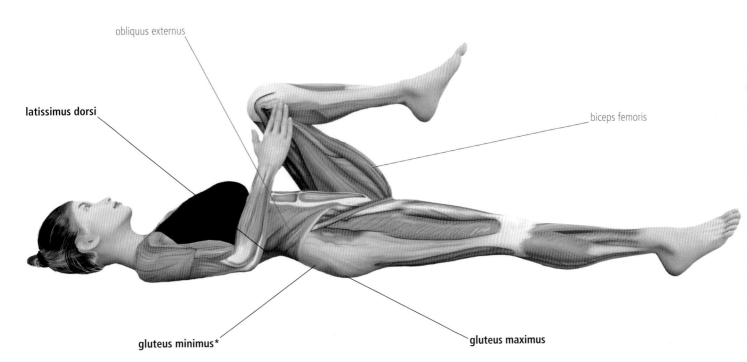

# UNILATERAL LEG RAISE

**①** Lie on your back with both legs extended and your spine in a imprinted position so that your lower back touches the floor.

**DO IT RIGHT**
• Slightly tuck your pelvis to help keep your spine grounded and your lower back on the floor.

**AVOID**
• Lifting your head or upper back.
• Holding your breath.

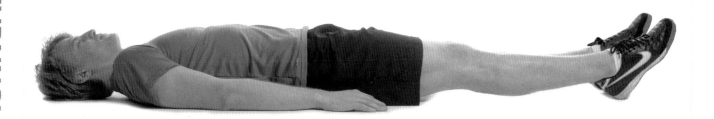

**TARGETS**
• Lower back
• Groin muscles
• Gluteal area
• Hamstrings

**LEVEL**
• Intermediate

**BENEFITS**
• Stretches lower back, hip extensors, and hip rotators

**NOT ADVISABLE IF YOU HAVE . . .**
• Advanced degenerative joint disease

**②** With your hands placed on your hamstrings just below the knee, extend and straighten your left leg toward the ceiling.

**③** Point both feet, and hold for 15 to 30 seconds.

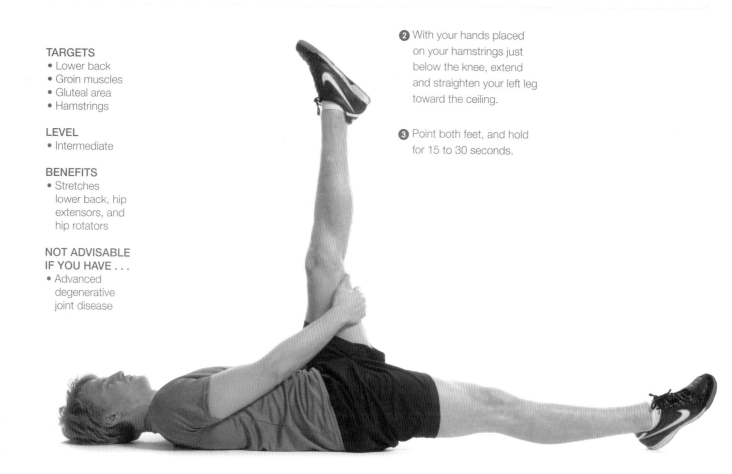

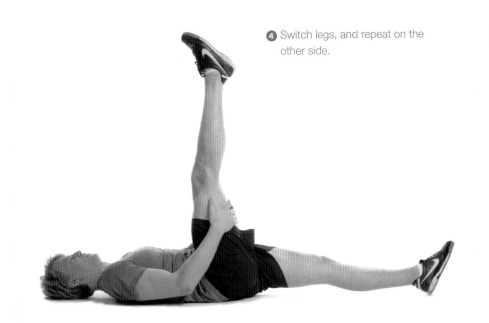

**4** Switch legs, and repeat on the other side.

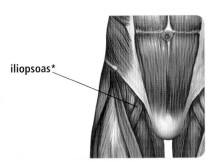

iliopsoas*

## BEST FOR

- erector spinae
- gluteus maximus
- gluteus medius
- gluteus minimus
- biceps femoris
- semitendinosus
- semimembranosus
- iliopsoas
- gastrocnemius
- soleus

**ANNOTATION KEY**

Black text indicates target muscles

* indicates deep muscles

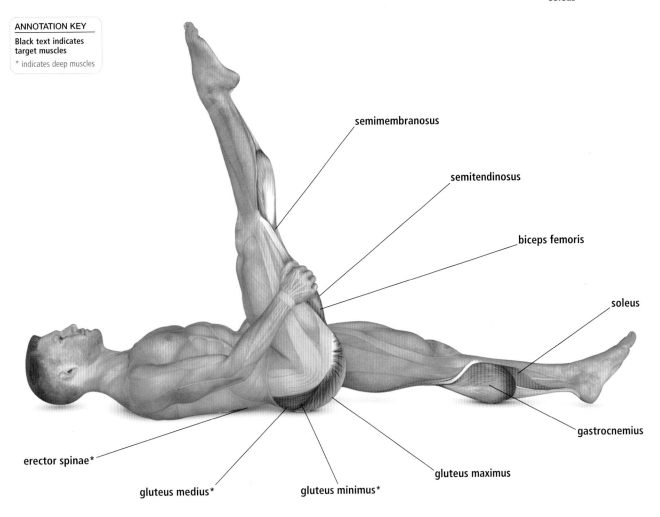

semimembranosus

semitendinosus

biceps femoris

soleus

gastrocnemius

erector spinae*

gluteus medius*

gluteus minimus*

gluteus maximus

# SUPINE FIGURE 4

**1** Lie on your back with your legs extended and toes pointed.

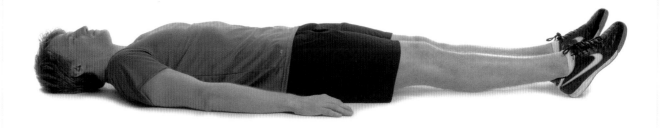

**2** Bend your right knee and turn the leg out so that your right ankle rests on your left thigh just above the knee, creating a figure 4.

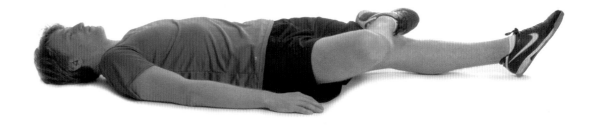

**TARGETS**
• Gluteal area

**LEVEL**
• Beginner

**BENEFITS**
• Stretches glutes and lower back

**NOT ADVISABLE IF YOU HAVE . . .**
• Knee issues
• Severe lower-back pain

**3** Bend your left leg, drawing both legs (still in the figure 4 position) in toward your chest as you grasp the back of your left thigh.

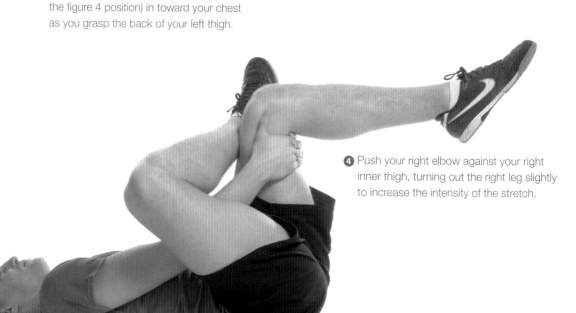

**4** Push your right elbow against your right inner thigh, turning out the right leg slightly to increase the intensity of the stretch.

**5** Return to the starting position, switch legs, and repeat.

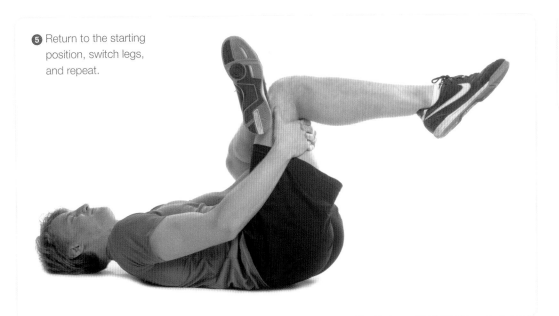

### DO IT RIGHT
- Keep your head and shoulder blades on the floor.
- Relax your hips so that you can go deeper into the stretch.
- Perform the stretch slowly.

### BEST FOR
- gluteus maximus
- gluteus medius
- gluteus minimus
- piriformis

### AVOID
- Twisting your lower body; instead—look for your hips to remain square.

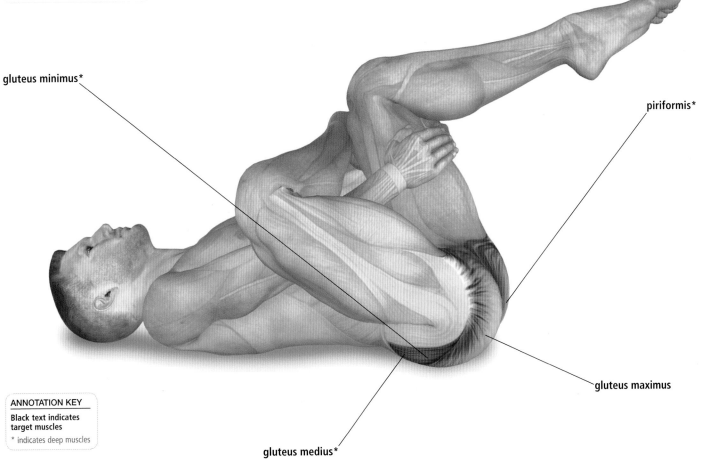

gluteus minimus*

piriformis*

gluteus maximus

gluteus medius*

**ANNOTATION KEY**

Black text indicates target muscles

* indicates deep muscles

# SIDE-LYING KNEE BEND

❶ Lie on your left side, with your legs extended together in line with your body. Extend your left arm, and rest your head on your upper arm.

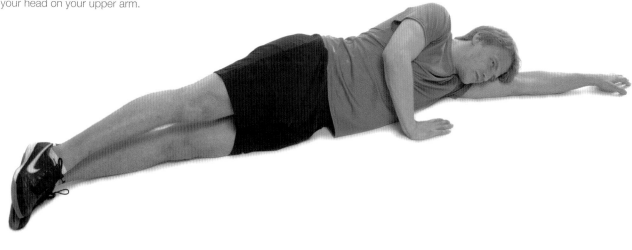

**TARGETS**
• Quadriceps

**LEVEL**
• Beginner

**BENEFITS**
• Helps to keep thigh muscles flexible

**NOT ADVISABLE IF YOU HAVE . . .**
• Knee issues

❷ Bend your right knee and grasp the ankle with your right hand.

❸ Pull your ankle in toward your buttocks as you stretch.

❹ Return to the starting position, and repeat on the other side.

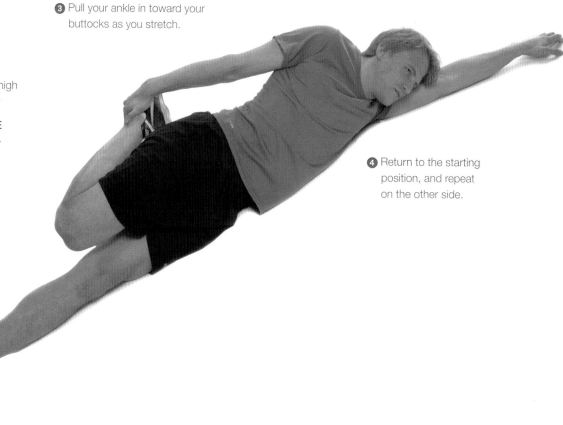

## DO IT RIGHT
- Keep your knees together, one on top of the other.
- Tuck your pelvis slightly forward and lift your chest to engage and stretch your core.
- Keep your foot pointed and parallel with your leg.

## AVOID
- Leaning back onto your gluteal muscles.
- Place a towel under your bottom hip if it feels uncomfortable to rest directly on the floor.

## BEST FOR
- rectus femoris
- vastus lateralis
- vastus intermedius
- vastus medialis

### ANNOTATION KEY
**Black text indicates target muscles**
\* indicates deep muscles

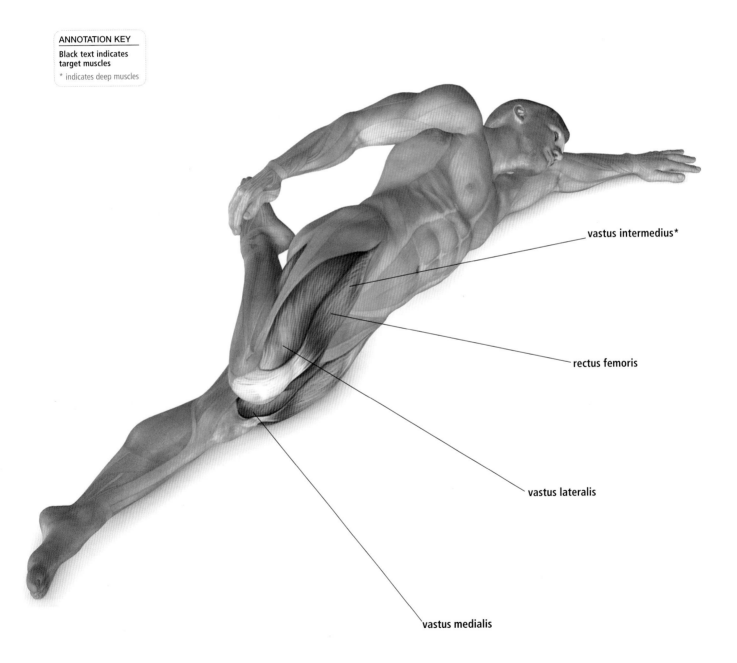

vastus intermedius*

rectus femoris

vastus lateralis

vastus medialis

# COBRA STRETCH

**1** Lie facedown, legs extended behind you with toes pointed. Position the palms of your hands on the floor slightly above your shoulders, and rest your elbows on the floor.

### DO IT RIGHT
- Lift out of your chest and back, rather than depending too much on your arms to create the arch in your back.
- Keep your shoulders and elbows pressed back to create more lift in your chest.
- Maintain pressure between the floor and your hips.

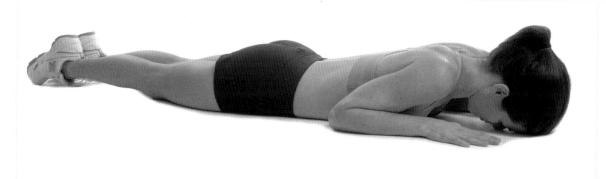

**2** Push down into the floor, and slowly lift through the top of your chest as you straighten your arms.

### TARGETS
- Abdominals
- Spinal joints

### LEVEL
- Intermediate

### BENEFITS
- Strengthens spine
- Stretches chest, abs, and shoulders

### NOT ADVISABLE IF YOU HAVE . . .
- Lower-back injury

**3** Pull your tailbone down toward your pubis as you push your shoulders down and back.

**4** Elongate your neck and gaze forward.

**5** Hold for up to 15 seconds. Release and repeat, performing three repetitions.

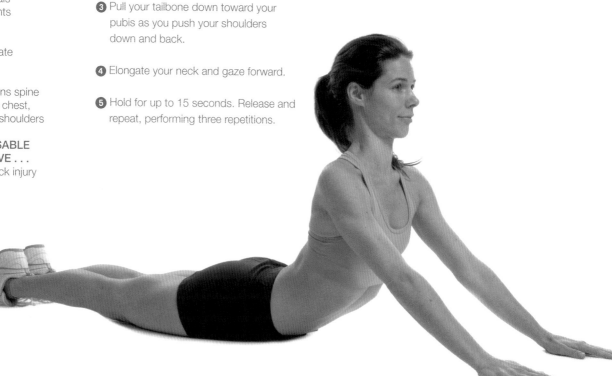

## AVOID

- Tensing your buttocks, which exerts pressure on your lower back.
- Splaying your elbows out to the sides.
- Lifting your hips off the floor.
- Tipping your head too far backward.
- Overdoing this stretch—it can lead to lower-back strain.

## MODIFICATION

**Easier:** Follow step 1, and then lift up out of your chest, bending your arms while keeping your hands flat on the floor close to your body.

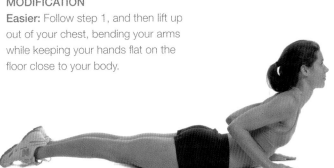

## BEST FOR

- erector spinae
- quadratus lumborum
- latissimus dorsi
- gluteus maximus
- gluteus medius
- pectoralis major
- rectus abdominis
- deltoideus medialis
- teres major
- teres minor

### ANNOTATION KEY

**Black text indicates target muscles**

Gray text indicates other working muscles

* indicates deep muscles

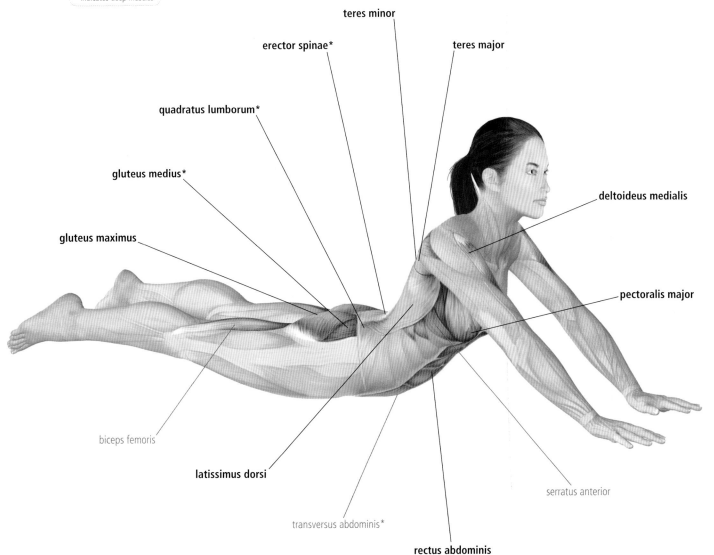

teres minor

erector spinae*

teres major

quadratus lumborum*

gluteus medius*

deltoideus medialis

gluteus maximus

pectoralis major

biceps femoris

latissimus dorsi

serratus anterior

transversus abdominis*

rectus abdominis

# SIDE-LYING RIB STRETCH

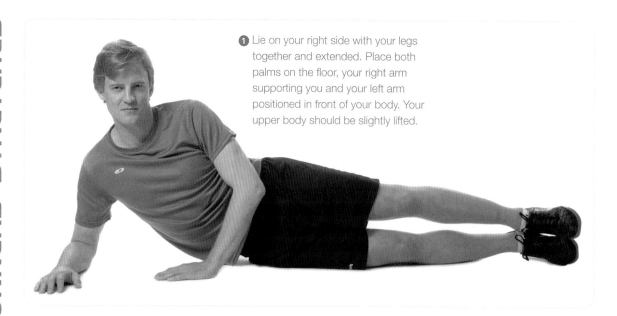

**1** Lie on your right side with your legs together and extended. Place both palms on the floor, your right arm supporting you and your left arm positioned in front of your body. Your upper body should be slightly lifted.

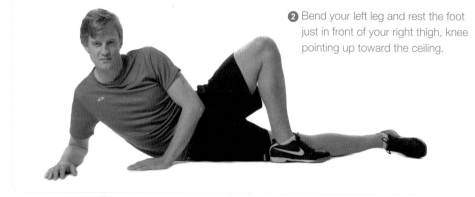

**2** Bend your left leg and rest the foot just in front of your right thigh, knee pointing up toward the ceiling.

**TARGETS**
• Rib cage
• Obliques
• Outer thighs
• Lower back

**LEVEL**
• Beginner

**BENEFITS**
• Strengthens lower back, obliques, and outer thighs

**NOT ADVISABLE IF YOU HAVE . . .**
• Severe lower-back pain

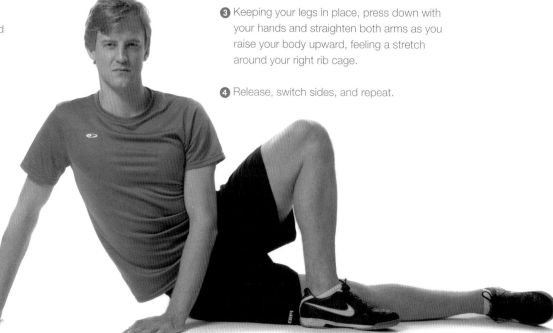

**3** Keeping your legs in place, press down with your hands and straighten both arms as you raise your body upward, feeling a stretch around your right rib cage.

**4** Release, switch sides, and repeat.

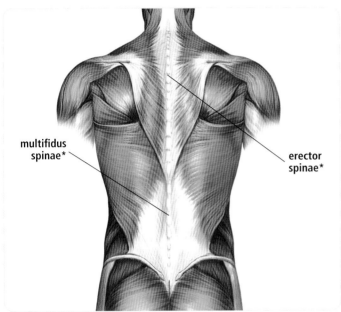

multifidus spinae*

erector spinae*

### DO IT RIGHT
- Shift your weight forward on your supporting hip.
- Place a towel under your bottom hip if you are uncomfortable resting directly on the floor.

### AVOID
- Tightening your jaw muscles, which can cause tension in your neck.

### BEST FOR
- obliquus externus
- obliquus internus
- tensor fasciae latae
- multifidus spinae
- erector spinae

### ANNOTATION KEY
Black text indicates target muscles
* indicates deep muscles

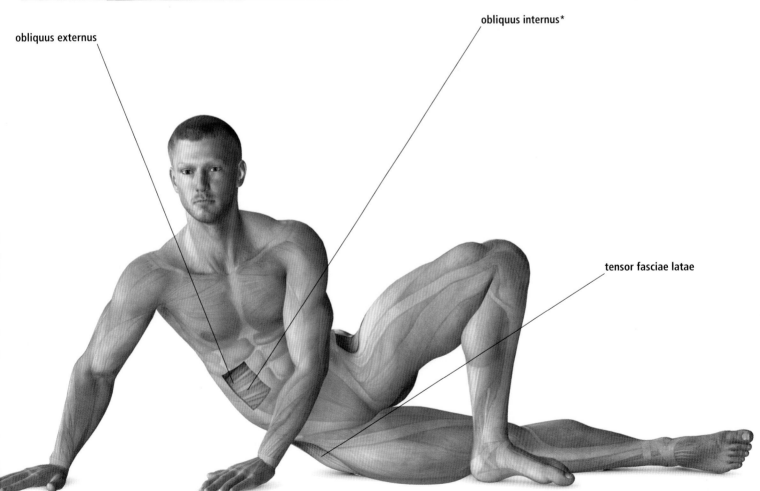

obliquus internus*

obliquus externus

tensor fasciae latae

# HIP/ILIOTIBIAL BAND STRETCH

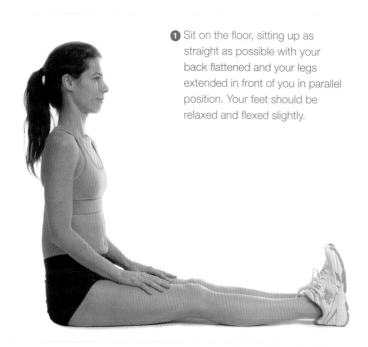

**1** Sit on the floor, sitting up as straight as possible with your back flattened and your legs extended in front of you in parallel position. Your feet should be relaxed and flexed slightly.

### DO IT RIGHT
- Keep your neck and shoulders relaxed.
- Apply even pressure to your leg with your active hand.
- Keep your torso upright as you pull your knee and torso together.

### AVOID
- Rounding your torso.
- Lifting the foot of your bent leg off the floor.
- Straining your neck as you rotate.

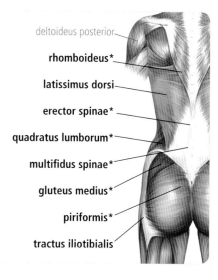

deltoideus posterior

**rhomboideus***

**latissimus dorsi**

**erector spinae***

**quadratus lumborum***

**multifidus spinae***

**gluteus medius***

**piriformis***

**tractus iliotibialis**

**2** Extend your left leg straight in front of you, and bend your right knee. Cross your bent knee over the straight leg, and keep your foot flat on the floor.

**3** Wrap your left arm around the bent knee so that you are able to apply pressure to your leg to rotate your torso.

### TARGETS
- Hips
- Gluteal area
- Spine
- Obliques

### LEVEL
- Intermediate

### BENEFITS
- Stretches hip extensors and flexors
- Stretches obliques

### NOT ADVISABLE IF YOU HAVE . . .
- Severe lower-back pain

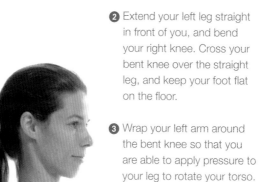

**4** Keeping your hips aligned, rotate your upper spine as you pull your chest in toward your knee.

**5** Hold for 30 seconds. Slowly release, and repeat three times on each side.

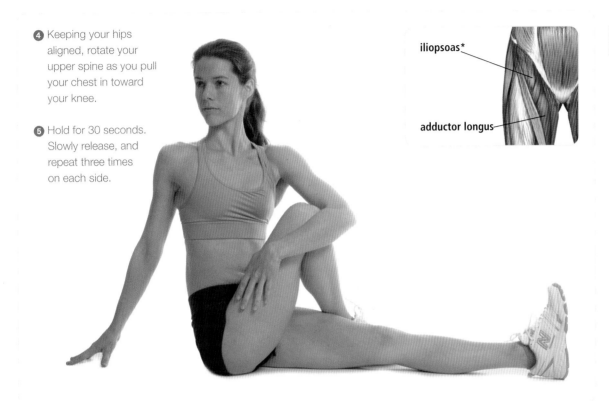

iliopsoas*

adductor longus

### BEST FOR

- adductor longus
- iliopsoas
- rhomboideus
- sternocleidomastoideus
- latissimus dorsi
- obliquus internus
- obliquus externus
- quadratus lumborum
- erector spinae
- multifidus spinae
- tractus iliotibialis
- gluteus maximus
- gluteus medius
- piriformis

### ANNOTATION KEY

**Black text indicates target muscles**

Gray text indicates other working muscles

\* indicates deep muscles

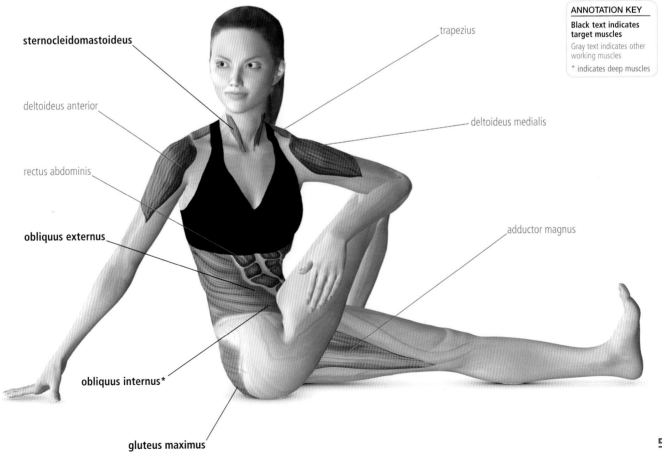

sternocleidomastoideus

trapezius

deltoideus anterior

rectus abdominis

deltoideus medialis

obliquus externus

adductor magnus

obliquus internus*

gluteus maximus

# PRETZEL STRETCH

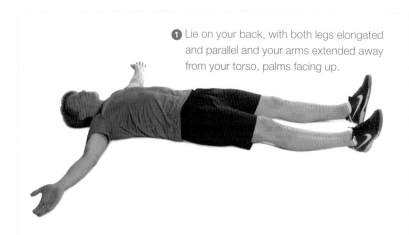

**1** Lie on your back, with both legs elongated and parallel and your arms extended away from your torso, palms facing up.

### DO IT RIGHT
- Keep your elbows and wrists lower than your shoulders, protecting your rotator cuff from strain.
- Before you cross one leg over the other, ensure that your body is in a straight line from your head to toe.

### AVOID
- Lifting your shoulders; try to keep both shoulder blades in contact with the floor throughout the stretch.

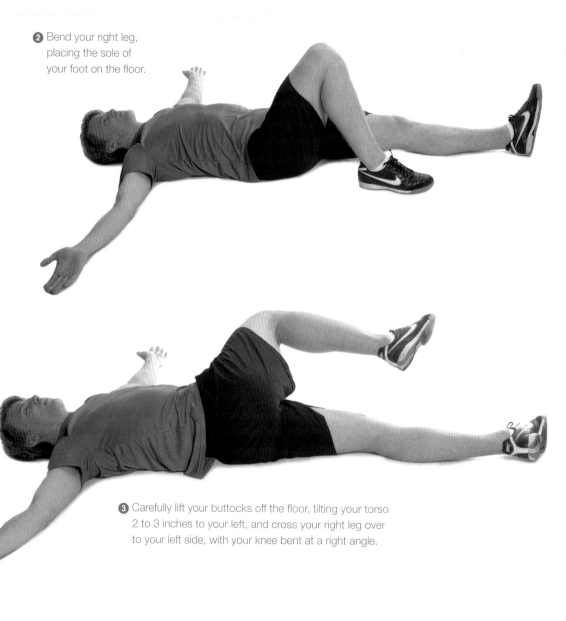

**2** Bend your right leg, placing the sole of your foot on the floor.

### TARGETS
- Lumbar spine
- Gluteal area
- Chest

### LEVEL
- Intermediate

### BENEFITS
- Stretches lower back

### NOT ADVISABLE IF YOU HAVE . . .
- Severe lower-back pain

**3** Carefully lift your buttocks off the floor, tilting your torso 2 to 3 inches to your left, and cross your right leg over to your left side, with your knee bent at a right angle.

**4** Hold, return to the starting position, and repeat on the other side.

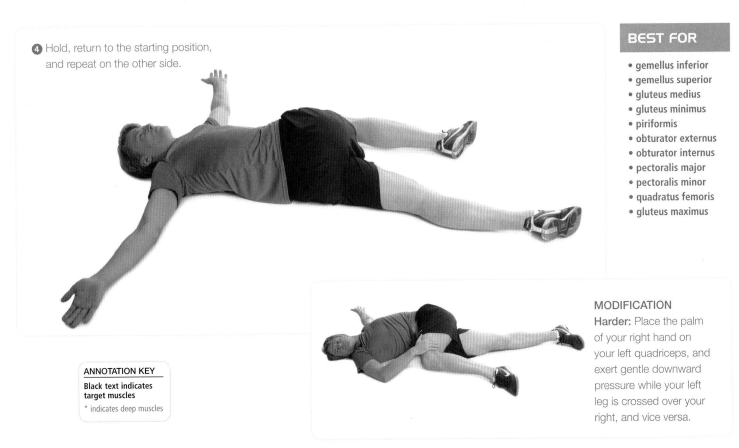

**BEST FOR**

- gemellus inferior
- gemellus superior
- gluteus medius
- gluteus minimus
- piriformis
- obturator externus
- obturator internus
- pectoralis major
- pectoralis minor
- quadratus femoris
- gluteus maximus

**MODIFICATION**

**Harder:** Place the palm of your right hand on your left quadriceps, and exert gentle downward pressure while your left leg is crossed over your right, and vice versa.

**ANNOTATION KEY**

**Black text indicates target muscles**

* indicates deep muscles

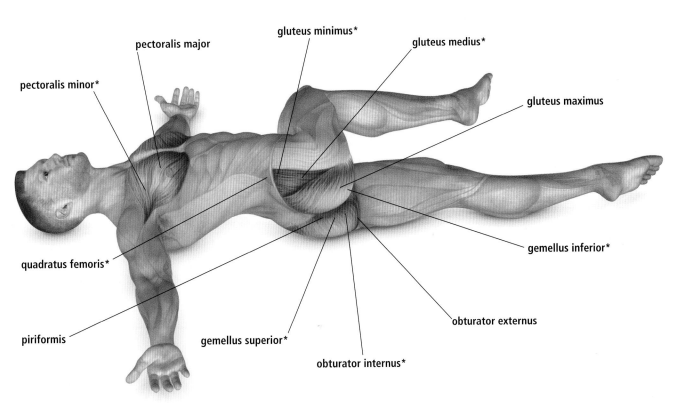

pectoralis minor*

pectoralis major

gluteus minimus*

gluteus medius*

gluteus maximus

gemellus inferior*

quadratus femoris*

obturator externus

piriformis

gemellus superior*

obturator internus*

# HEEL-DROP/TOE-UP STRETCH

### HEEL-DROP

**①** Stand on an aerobic step, a riser, or a stair with your legs and feet parallel and shoulder-width apart. Bend your knees very slightly and tuck your pelvis slightly forward, lift your chest, and press your shoulders downward and back.

**②** Position your left foot slightly in front of your right, and place the ball of your right foot on the edge of the step.

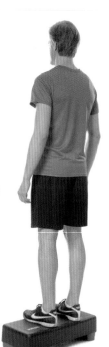

### AVOID
• Bouncing to achieve a greater stretch—all of your movements should be performed slowly and carefully.

**③** Drop your right heel down while controlling the amount of weight on the right leg to increase or decrease the intensity of the stretch in the right calf.

**④** Release, switch feet, and repeat on the other side.

### TARGETS
• Calves
• Achilles tendon

### LEVEL
• Beginner

### BENEFITS
• Stretches calf muscles and Achilles tendon

### NOT ADVISABLE IF YOU HAVE . . .
• Strained calf muscle

### DO IT RIGHT
• Use the wall or other stable object to balance yourself if necessary.
• Engage each head of your calf muscles by gently and slowly rolling from your big toe to your small toe and back again, shifting your body weight over your toes as you go.

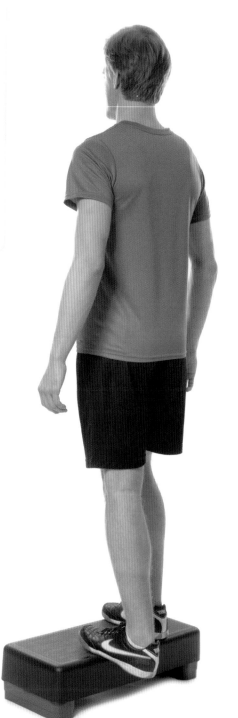

**TOE-UP**

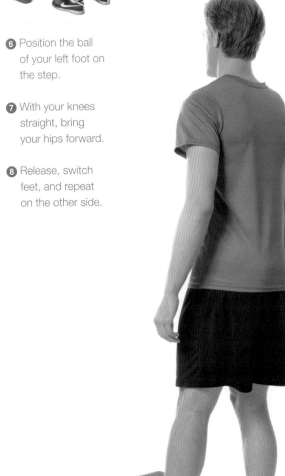

❺ Step down from the riser, and stand with your legs and feet parallel and shoulder-width apart. Bend your knees very slightly and tuck your pelvis slightly forward, lift your chest, and press your shoulders downward and back.

❻ Position the ball of your left foot on the step.

❼ With your knees straight, bring your hips forward.

❽ Release, switch feet, and repeat on the other side.

## BEST FOR

• gastrocnemius
• soleus
• tendo calcaneus

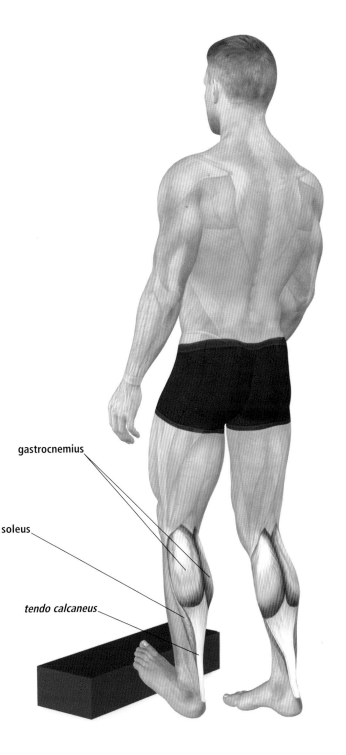

gastrocnemius

soleus

*tendo calcaneus*

# GASTROCNEMIUS STRETCH

**1** Stand with your legs straight, one foot behind the other.

**2** Bring your front leg forward and bend your front knee.

**3** Keeping both heels on the floor, lean into your front leg until you feel the stretch in your back calf muscle. Hold for 15 seconds. Repeat sequence three times on each leg.

**DO IT RIGHT**
• Keep your chest upright and lifted as you lean into the stretch.

**TARGETS**
• Calves

**LEVEL**
• Beginner

**BENEFITS**
• Stretches gastrocnemius muscle

**NOT ADVISABLE IF YOU HAVE . . .**
• Strained calf muscle

**BEST FOR**

• **gastrocnemius**

**AVOID**
• Bending your extended leg.
• Lifting your heel off the floor.

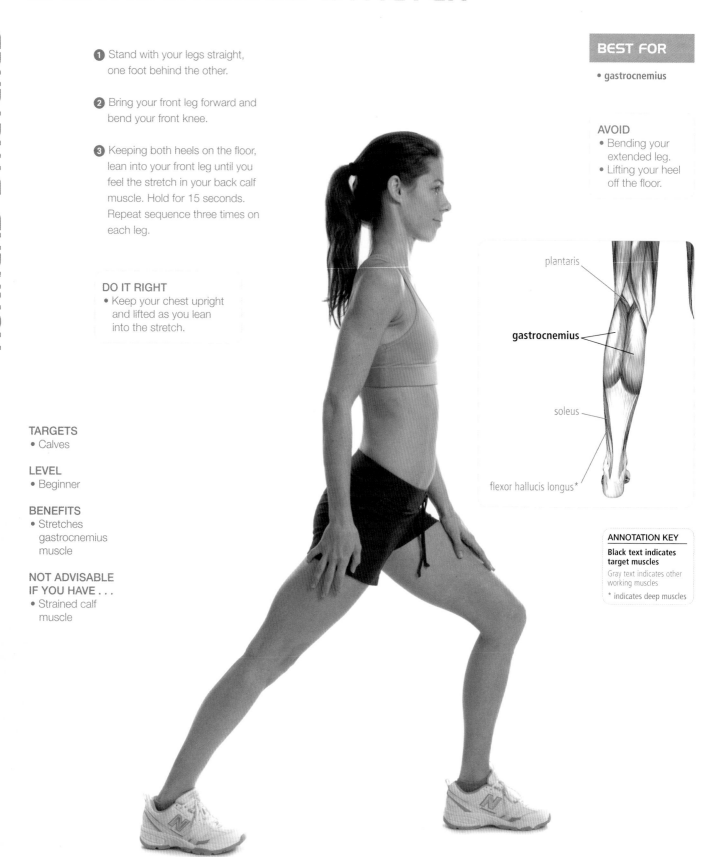

plantaris

**gastrocnemius**

soleus

flexor hallucis longus*

**ANNOTATION KEY**

**Black text indicates target muscles**

Gray text indicates other working muscles

* indicates deep muscles

# SOLEUS STRETCH

1. Stand with one foot about one stride length back, knee bent.

2. Bring the other foot forward and bend at the knee.

3. Keeping both heels on the floor, lean into the stretch as you bend your back knee. Once you feel the stretch, hold the position for 15 seconds. Repeat stretch three times. Switch legs and repeat sequence three times.

**DO IT RIGHT**
- Keep your chest upright and lifted as you lean into the stretch.

**AVOID**
- Lifting your heel off the floor.

**BEST FOR**
- soleus

**TARGETS**
- Calves

**LEVEL**
- Beginner

**BENEFITS**
- Stretches soleus muscle

**NOT ADVISABLE IF YOU HAVE . . .**
- Strained calf muscle

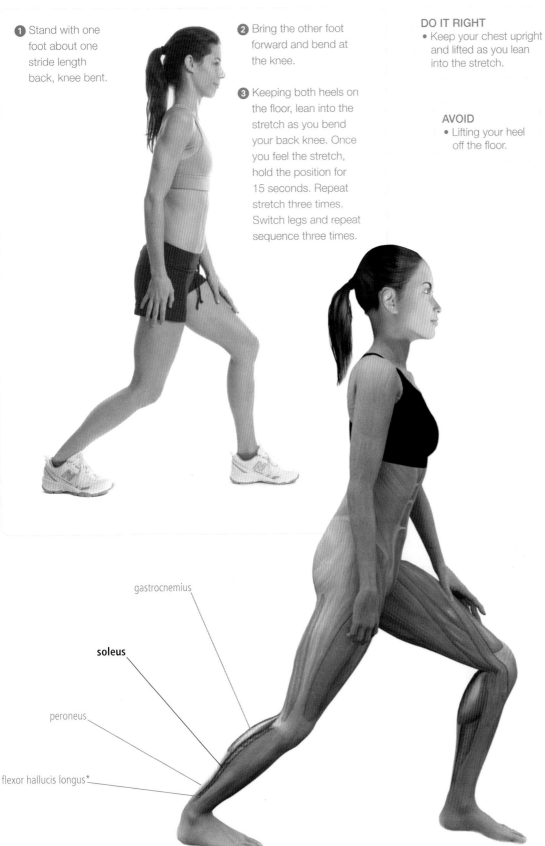

gastrocnemius

soleus

peroneus

flexor hallucis longus*

**ANNOTATION KEY**
**Black text indicates target muscles**
Gray text indicates other working muscles
* indicates deep muscles

# ILIOTIBIAL BAND STRETCH

**1** Standing, cross your left leg in front of your right.

**2** Bend forward from the hips while keeping both legs straight, and reach your hands toward the floor.

**3** Hold for 15 seconds. Repeat the sequence three times on each leg.

## BEST FOR

- tractus iliotibialis
- biceps femoris
- gluteus maximus
- vastus lateralis

**TARGETS**
- Iliotibial band
- Hamstrings

**LEVEL**
- Beginner

**BENEFITS**
- Helps to stabilize knee joints
- Helps to keep hips flexible
- Stretches back, hamstrings, and calves

**NOT ADVISABLE IF YOU HAVE . . .**
- Neck issues
- Lower-back pain

**AVOID**
- Raising your back heel off the floor.
- Arching or round your back.

**DO IT RIGHT**
- Keep both feet flat on the floor.
- Stretch with good alignment so that your back leg and your spine form a straight line

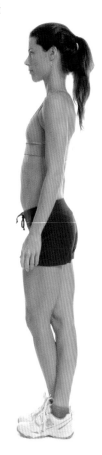

tractus iliotibialis

gluteus maximus

biceps femoris

rectus femoris

semitendinosus

semimembranosus

vastus lateralis

gastrocnemius

soleus

**ANNOTATION KEY**

**Black text indicates target muscles**

Gray text indicates other working muscles

# RESISTANCE BAND TENDON STRETCH

**1** Grasp a resistance band with an end in each hand, and loop it around the bottom of your right foot. Lie on your back with your left leg extended and your spine in a imprinted position so that your lower back touches the floor. Keep your right leg elevated only high enough to maintain tension in the band.

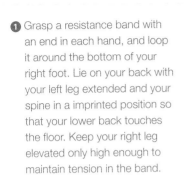

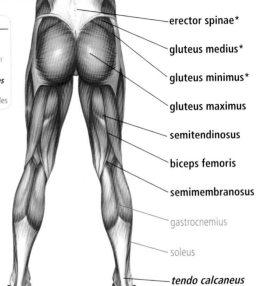

**ANNOTATION KEY**

**Black text indicates target muscles**

Gray text indicates other working muscles

*Black italics indicates tendons*

\* indicates deep muscles

erector spinae*
gluteus medius*
gluteus minimus*
gluteus maximus
semitendinosus
biceps femoris
semimembranosus
gastrocnemius
soleus
*tendo calcaneus*

**2** Pull the band toward your chest with both hands so you extend and straighten your right leg toward the ceiling to a 90-degree angle.

**3** Hold for 15 to 30 seconds, and then switch legs, and repeat on the other side.

**DO IT RIGHT**
• Keep even tension in both hands.
• Keep your elevated leg straight.

**AVOID**
• Lifting or bending the leg extended on the floor.

**BEST FOR**

• biceps femoris
• semitendinosus
• semimembranosus
• erector spinae
• gluteus maximus
• gluteus medius
• gluteus minimus
• tendo calcaneus

**TARGETS**
• Hamstrings
• Gluteal area
• Achilles tendon

**LEVEL**
• Intermediate

**BENEFITS**
• Stretches lower back, hip extensors, and hip rotators

**NOT ADVISABLE IF YOU HAVE . . .**
• Advanced degenerative joint disease

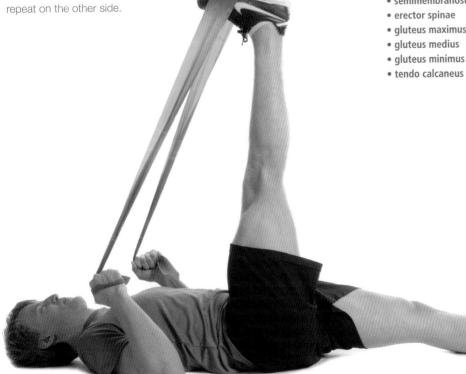

# RESISTANCE BAND ANKLE STRETCHES

**1** Sit on a chair with your feet flat on the floor.

**2** Loop an elastic exercise band around your right foot, and then take hold of both ends of the band with your right hand.

**3** Keeping your right leg stable, point your right foot and pull the band to the right, stretching the inside of the ankle.

**AVOID**
- Shifting your weight to the side while you are stretching; your weight should be evenly balanced on your sitting bones.

**DO IT RIGHT**
- Use a towel if you don't have an elastic resistance band.

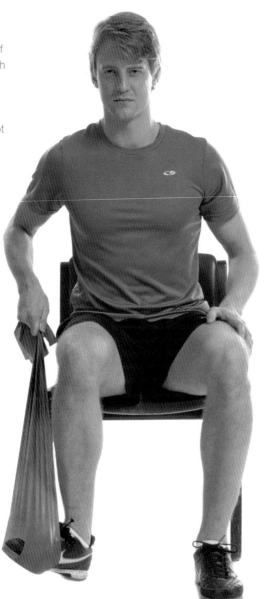

**TARGETS**
- Ankles

**LEVEL**
- Beginner

**BENEFITS**
- Stretches ankles, calves, and shins

**NOT ADVISABLE IF YOU HAVE . . .**
- Acute ankle pain

**BEST FOR**
- peroneus longus
- peroneus brevis
- tibialis anterior

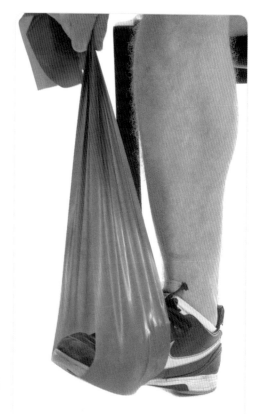

**PERONEUS STRETCH**

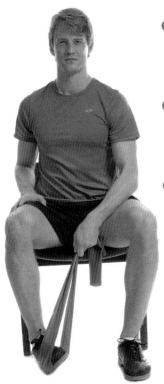

④ Keeping the band looped around your right foot, transfer both ends of the band to your left hand.

⑤ Keeping your right leg stable, point your right foot and pull the band to the left, stretching the outside of the ankle.

⑥ Switch legs, and repeat both stretches on the other side.

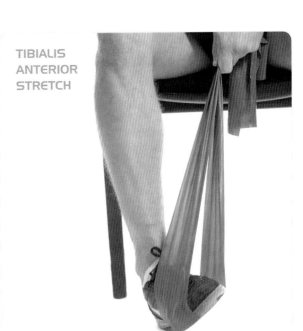

**TIBIALIS ANTERIOR STRETCH**

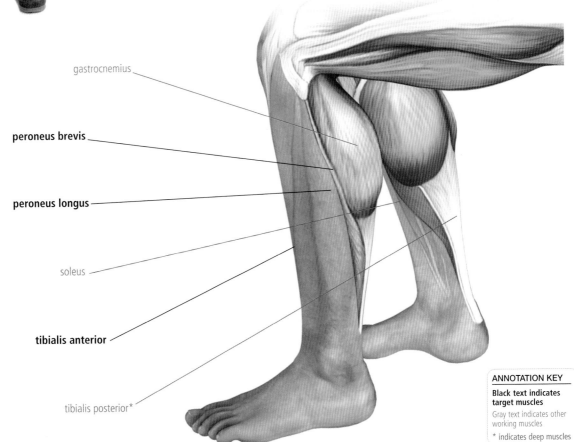

gastrocnemius

**peroneus brevis**

**peroneus longus**

soleus

**tibialis anterior**

tibialis posterior*

**ANNOTATION KEY**

**Black text indicates target muscles**

Gray text indicates other working muscles

* indicates deep muscles

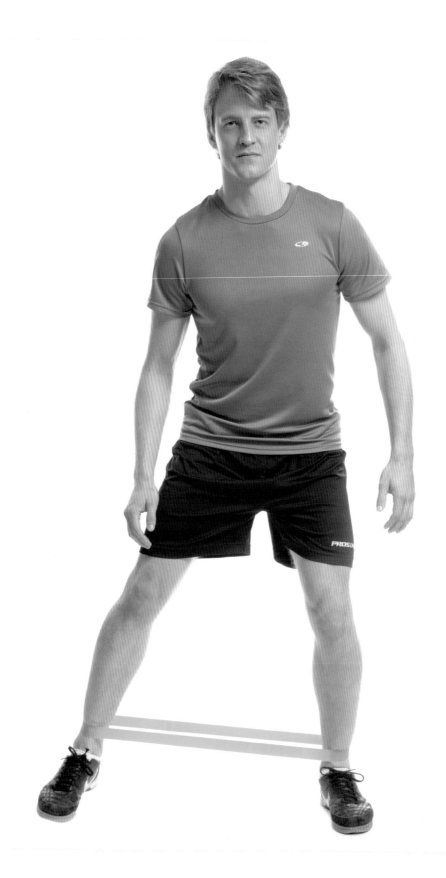

# TARGET: PRIMARY MUSCLES

Your body calls on a few large muscle groups to run: your quadriceps, hamstrings, gluteals, and psoas. The large quadriceps femoris group (rectus femoris, vastus lateralis, vastus intermedius, and vastus medialis) is located at the front of the thigh; located on the back of the thigh, the biceps femoris, semitendinosus, and semimembranosus make up the group known as the hamstrings. The largest muscle in your body—the gluteus maximus—really comes into play only when you run, along with the gluteus medius and gluteus minimus. The last of the primary running muscles is the iliopsoas (also known as the psoas major and iliacus).

The following exercises target these large antagonist and agonist muscles, which work in concert to move and stabilize you. An antagonist pair consists of an extensor muscle, such as the gluteus maximus, which "opens" the hip joint, and a flexor, such as the iliopsoas, which does the opposite. Keeping them in proper balance (size, strength, and elasticity) is crucial to avoid injury and increase performance levels.

# DUMBBELL DEADLIFT

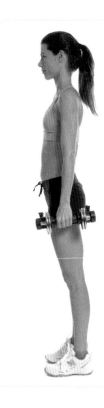

**1** Stand upright, feet planted about shoulder-width apart, with your arms slightly in front of your thighs with a hand weight or dumbbell in each hand. Your knees should be slightly bent and your rear pushed slightly outward.

## DO IT RIGHT
- Maintain the straight line of your back.
- Keep your torso stable.
- Keep your neck straight.
- Keep your arms extended.

## AVOID
- Allowing your lower back to sag or arch.
- Straining to look forward while you are bent over.

## TARGETS
- Hamstrings
- Back
- Gluteal area

## LEVEL
- Intermediate

## BENEFITS
- Improves flexibility
- Stabilizes lower body

## NOT ADVISABLE IF YOU HAVE . . .
- Lower-back pain

**2** Keeping your back flat, hinge at the hips and bend forward as you lower the dumbbells toward the floor. You should feel a stretch in the backs of your legs.

**3** With control, raise your upper body back to starting position. Repeat, completing three sets of 15.

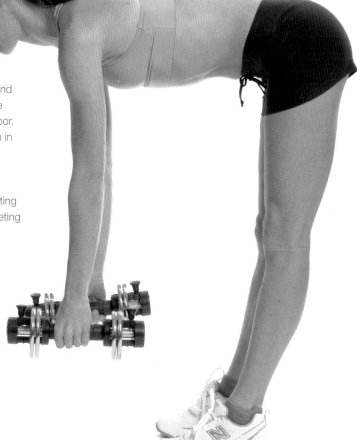

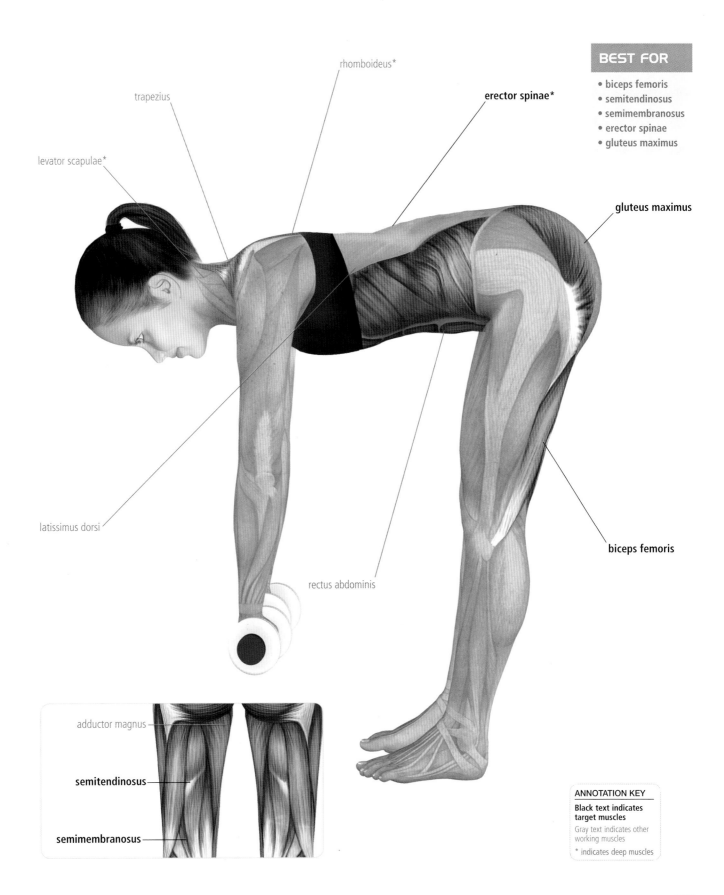

rhomboideus*

trapezius

erector spinae*

**BEST FOR**
- biceps femoris
- semitendinosus
- semimembranosus
- erector spinae
- gluteus maximus

levator scapulae*

**gluteus maximus**

latissimus dorsi

**biceps femoris**

rectus abdominis

adductor magnus

**semitendinosus**

**semimembranosus**

**ANNOTATION KEY**

**Black text indicates
target muscles**

Gray text indicates other
working muscles

* indicates deep muscles

# HIP EXTENSION AND FLEXION

**❶** Stand with your feet shoulder-width apart, with a resistance loop or a resistance band tied around your ankles. Tuck your pelvis slightly forward, lift your chest, and press your shoulders downward and back.

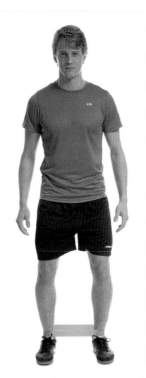

**❷** Keeping your head up, shoulders back, place your hands on your hips, slowly extend your leg backward.

**❸** Perform three sets of 10 repetitions, and return to the starting position.

### AVOID
• Bending your knee.
• Allowing your hips to shift out of line.

### TARGETS
• Hip extensors
• Hip flexors

### LEVEL
• Beginner

### BENEFITS
• Strengthens hips

### NOT ADVISABLE IF YOU HAVE . . .
• Balance issues

### MODIFICATION
**Easier:** Complete steps 1 through 5, holding onto a support such as a mop handle or chair back.

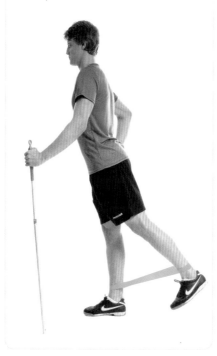

**HIP EXTENSION**

### DO IT RIGHT
• Tighten your glutes as you move your leg backward during the extension phase of the exercise
• Tighten the muscles at the front of your thigh and hip as you move your leg forward during the flexion phase of the exercise.

**4** Keeping your back and knee straight, slowly extend your leg forward.

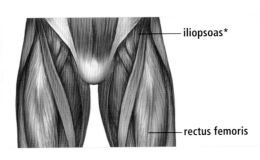

iliopsoas*

rectus femoris

## BEST FOR

- rectus femoris
- iliopsoas
- gluteus maximus
- biceps femoris
- semitendinosus
- semimembranosus

**5** Perform three sets of 10 repetitions, return to the starting position, and repeat entire sequence on the opposite side.

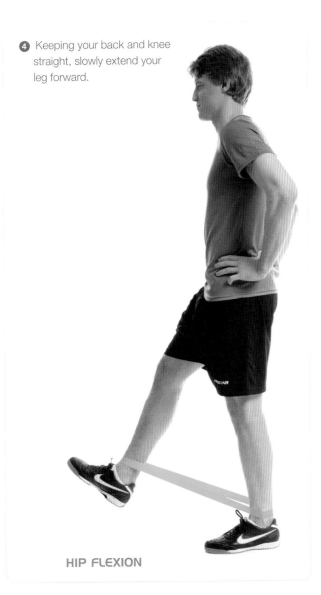

HIP FLEXION

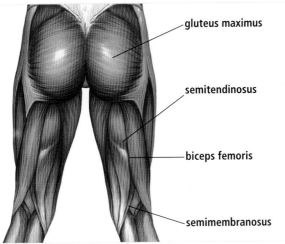

gluteus maximus

semitendinosus

biceps femoris

semimembranosus

ANNOTATION KEY

**Black text indicates target muscles**

* indicates deep muscles

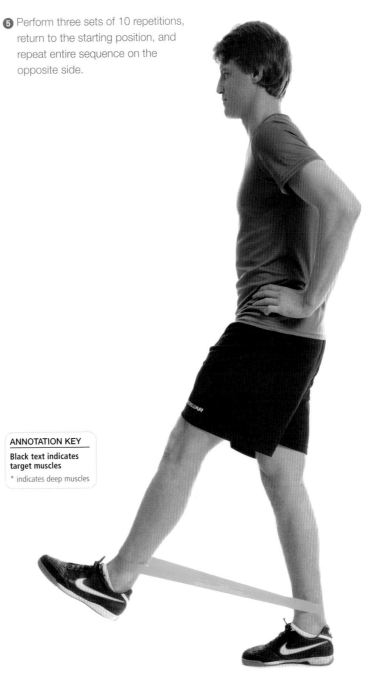

# HIP ABDUCTION AND ADDUCTION

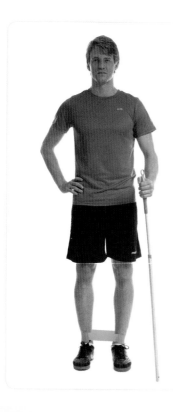

1. Stand with your feet shoulder-width apart, with a resistance loop or a resistance band tied around your ankles. Tuck your pelvis slightly forward, lift your chest, and press your shoulders downward and back. With your left hand, hold onto a support such as a mop handle or chair back.

2. Keeping your back and knee straight and foot facing forward, move your right foot directly to the right, moving away from your body. Hold for 2 seconds and repeat 10 times.

3. Return to starting position.

**TARGETS**
- Hip abductors
- Hip adductors

**LEVEL**
- Beginner

**BENEFITS**
- Strengthens hips

**NOT ADVISABLE IF YOU HAVE . . .**
- Balance issues

**DO IT RIGHT**
- Tighten the muscles at the side of your thigh and hip as you move your leg.

**AVOID**
- Touching your moving foot to the floor as you move your foot sideways and inward.
- Leaning your torso to one side.

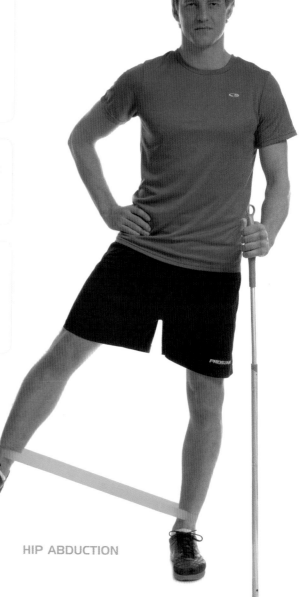

HIP ABDUCTION

4 Keeping your back and knee straight and foot facing forward, move your left foot directly to the right, moving it toward and across your body. Hold for 2 seconds and repeat 10 times.

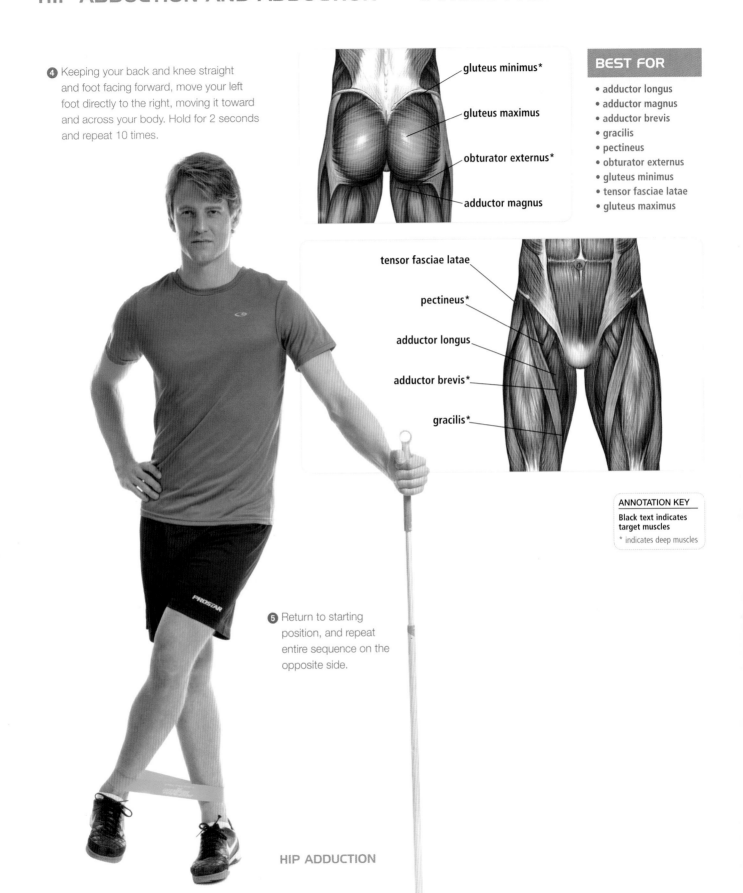

gluteus minimus*

gluteus maximus

obturator externus*

adductor magnus

tensor fasciae latae

pectineus*

adductor longus

adductor brevis*

gracilis*

**BEST FOR**

- adductor longus
- adductor magnus
- adductor brevis
- gracilis
- pectineus
- obturator externus
- gluteus minimus
- tensor fasciae latae
- gluteus maximus

**ANNOTATION KEY**

Black text indicates target muscles

* indicates deep muscles

5 Return to starting position, and repeat entire sequence on the opposite side.

HIP ADDUCTION

# SIDE STEPS

**1** Stand with your feet shoulder-width apart, with a resistance loop or a resistance band tied around your ankles. Tuck your pelvis slightly forward, lift your chest, and press your shoulders downward and back.

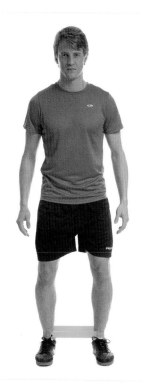

**TARGETS**
• Hip adductors

**LEVEL**
• Beginner

**BENEFITS**
• Strengthens hips

**NOT ADVISABLE
IF YOU HAVE . . .**
• Acute hip pain

**2** Keeping your head up, shoulders back, place your hands on your hips, and step sideways as far as you can while keeping your knees slightly bent and your posture tall.

**AVOID**
• Leaning your torso to one side.

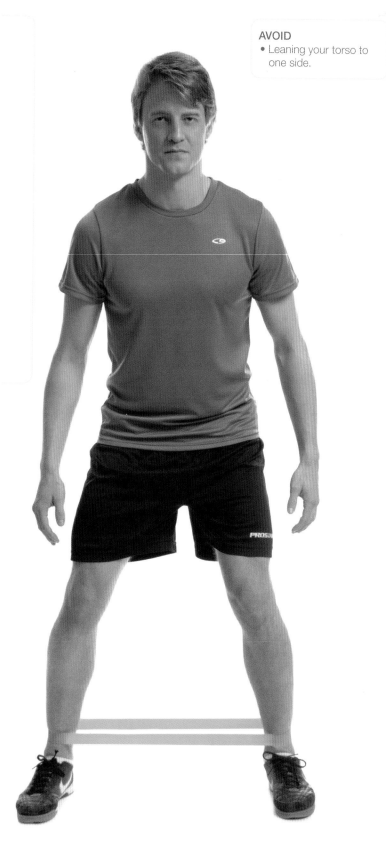

**DO IT RIGHT**
• Tighten the muscles at the side of your thigh and hip as you move your leg.

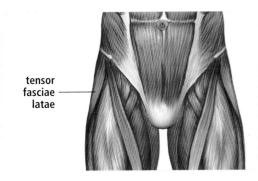

tensor
fasciae
latae

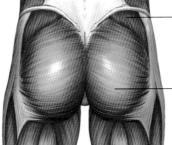

gluteus
minimus*

gluteus
maximus

**BEST FOR**

- gluteus minimus*
- tensor fasciae latae
- gluteus maximus

**ANNOTATION KEY**

**Black text indicates target muscles**

* indicates deep muscles

**③** Bring the opposite foot inward to meet the other foot, moving slowly and under control.

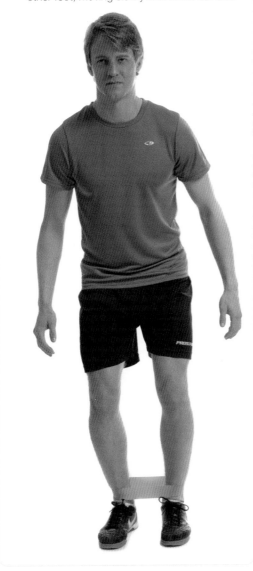

**④** Continue to step to the side for one to three sets of 8 to 12 repetitions, then repeat in the other direction.

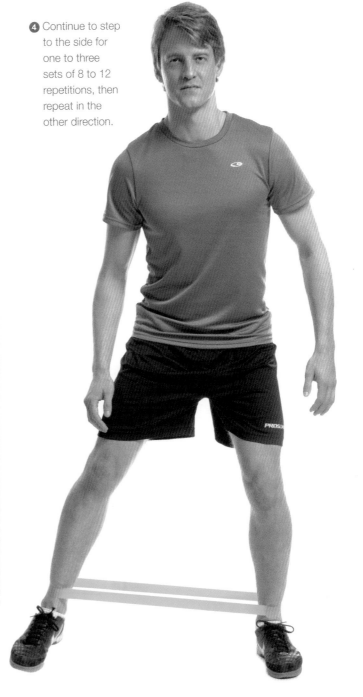

# CROSSOVER STEPS

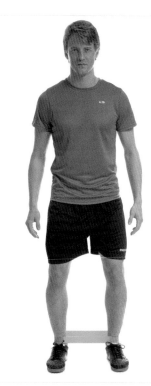

**1** Stand with your feet shoulder-width apart, with a resistance loop or a resistance band tied around your ankles. Tuck your pelvis slightly forward, lift your chest, and press your shoulders downward and back.

**DO IT RIGHT**
- Flex the toes of your moving foot toward your shin.
- Keep your hips square and pointed forward.
- Move at a pace that allows you to keep tension in the resistance band.

**TARGETS**
- Hip adductors

**LEVEL**
- Beginner

**BENEFITS**
- Strengthens hips

**NOT ADVISABLE IF YOU HAVE . . .**
- Acute hip pain

**2** Step out with your left foot until you feel moderate tension in the band, and then cross your left foot over your right.

**AVOID**
- Rotating your torso.
- Hunching your shoulders.

74

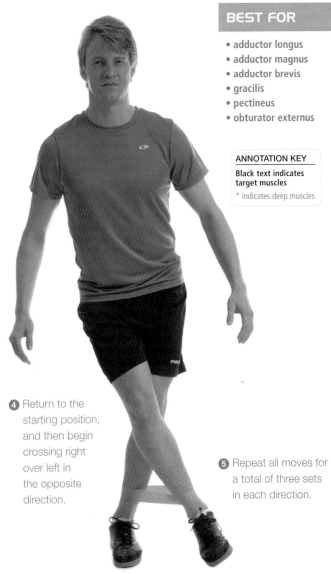

obturator externus*

adductor magnus

**3** Next, step your right foot in front of your left, and then step your left foot out, for a total of three steps with both feet to the left.

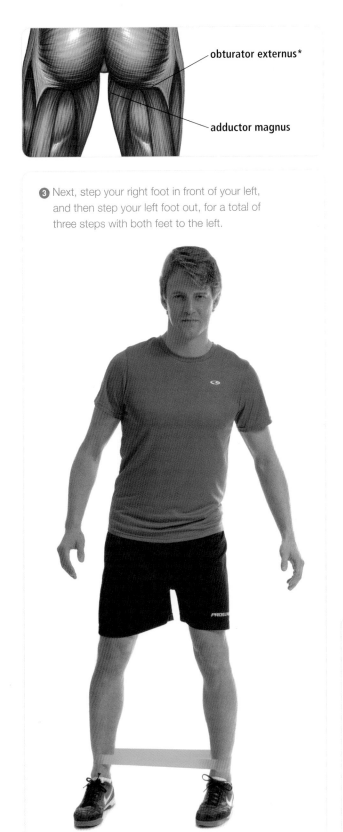

**4** Return to the starting position, and then begin crossing right over left in the opposite direction.

**5** Repeat all moves for a total of three sets in each direction.

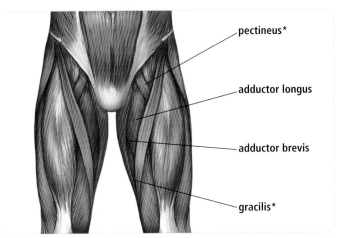

pectineus*

adductor longus

adductor brevis

gracilis*

# KNEE SQUAT

**1** Stand with your legs and feet parallel and shoulder-width apart, and your knees bent very slightly. Tuck your pelvis slightly forward, lift your chest, and press your shoulders down and back.

## DO IT RIGHT
- Keep your chest upright.
- Pull your abdominals in toward your spine.
- Curl your toes upward throughout the movement.
- Imagine pressing into the floor as you rise from the squat, creating your body's own resistance in your leg muscles.

## AVOID
- Allowing your heels to lift off the floor.
- Rising too quickly to the standing position.

## TARGETS
- Calves
- Arches of feet

## LEVEL
- Beginner

## BENEFITS
- Lengthens and strengthens calf muscles
- Improves balance

## NOT ADVISABLE IF YOU HAVE . . .
- Foot pain

**2** Extend your arms in front of your body for stability, keeping them even with your shoulders. With your feet planted firmly on the floor, curl your toes slightly upward.

**3** Draw in your abdominal muscles and bend into a squat. Keep your heels planted on the floor and your chest as upright as possible, resisting the urge to bend too far forward.

**4** Exhale, and return to the original position. Repeat five to six times.

**MODIFICATION**
**Harder:** Grasp a weighted medicine ball in both hands, and then follow steps 1 though 4.

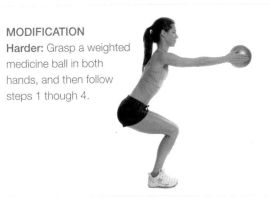

**MODIFICATION**
**Harder:** Secure a resistance band under both feet. Stand with feet shoulder-width apart, and then with an end in each hand, bring your hands to shoulder level. Perform steps 3 and 4.

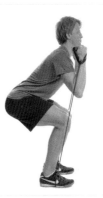

**BEST FOR**

- biceps femoris
- rectus femoris
- tibialis anterior
- gastrocnemius
- soleus
- gluteus maximus
- abductor hallucis
- vastus medialis

**ANNOTATION KEY**

**Black text indicates target muscles**
Gray text indicates other working muscles
* indicates deep muscles

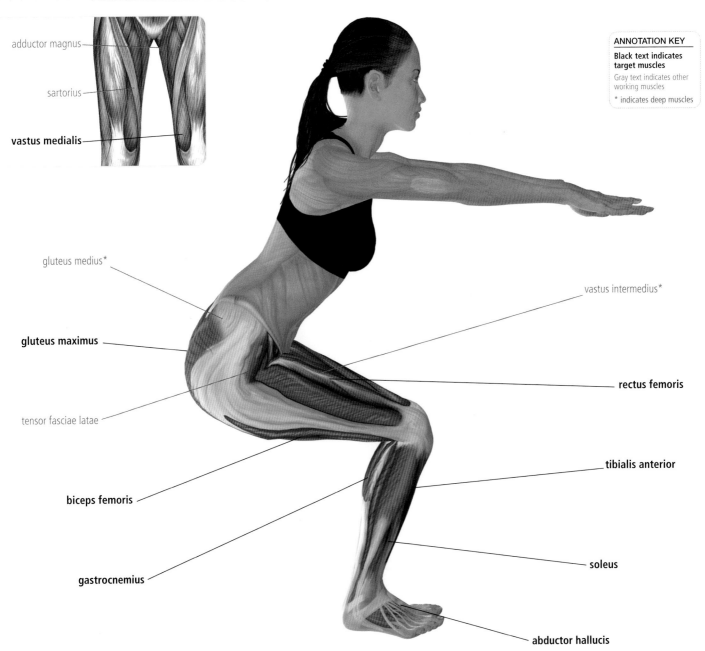

adductor magnus

sartorius

**vastus medialis**

gluteus medius*

**gluteus maximus**

tensor fasciae latae

**biceps femoris**

**gastrocnemius**

vastus intermedius*

**rectus femoris**

**tibialis anterior**

**soleus**

**abductor hallucis**

# SWISS BALL LOOP EXTENSION

**1** With a resistance loop or a resistance band tied around your ankles, lie prone on a Swiss ball, with your hips over the center of the ball as you support your weight on your arms. Your hands should be directly below your shoulders.

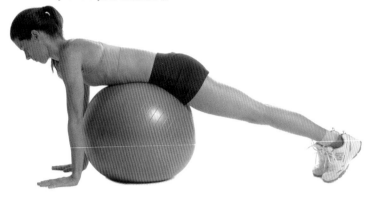

**DO IT RIGHT**
- Keep your hips in line with your shoulders and ankles to achieve optimal weight distribution.
- Keep your neck elongated and relaxed.
- Keep your core tight and your back flat.

**2** Keeping your abs tight, exhale, and squeeze your gluteal muscles to raise your right leg, lengthening your body as your weight transfers from your arms to your left foot, stretching through your heel.

**3** Return your right foot to the floor. Repeat 10 leg extensions on that side, holding a straight plank position throughout the exercise.

**TARGETS**
- Hip extensors
- Abdominal muscles
- Hamstrings

**LEVEL**
- Intermediate

**BENEFITS**
- Strengthens abs
- Strengthens hips and hamstrings

**NOT ADVISABLE IF YOU HAVE . . .**
- Shoulder issues

**AVOID**
- Allowing your shoulders to sink.

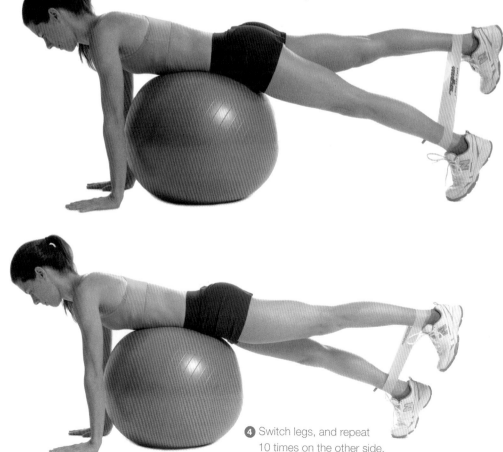

**4** Switch legs, and repeat 10 times on the other side.

# SWISS BALL LOOP EXTENSION • TARGET: PRIMARY MUSCLES

## MODIFICATION

**Advanced:** With a resistance loop or a resistance band tied around your ankles, prop your forearms on a Swiss ball, and then follow steps 1 through 4.

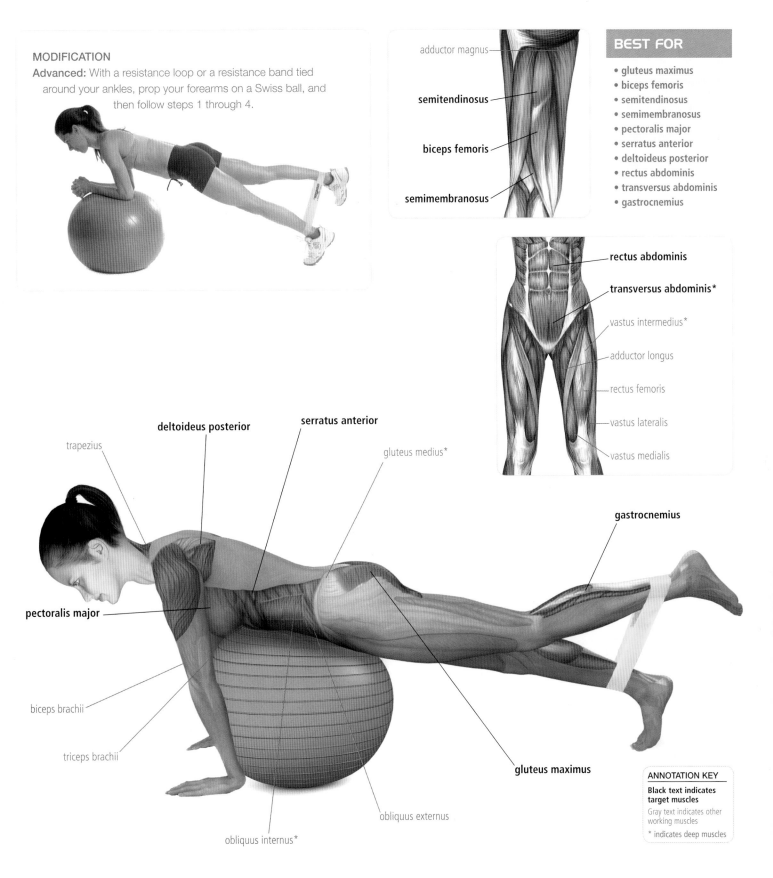

adductor magnus

semitendinosus

biceps femoris

semimembranosus

rectus abdominis

transversus abdominis*

vastus intermedius*

adductor longus

rectus femoris

vastus lateralis

vastus medialis

deltoideus posterior

serratus anterior

trapezius

gluteus medius*

gastrocnemius

pectoralis major

biceps brachii

triceps brachii

gluteus maximus

obliquus internus*

obliquus externus

**ANNOTATION KEY**

**Black text indicates target muscles**

Gray text indicates other working muscles

* indicates deep muscles

# PLANK LEG EXTENSION

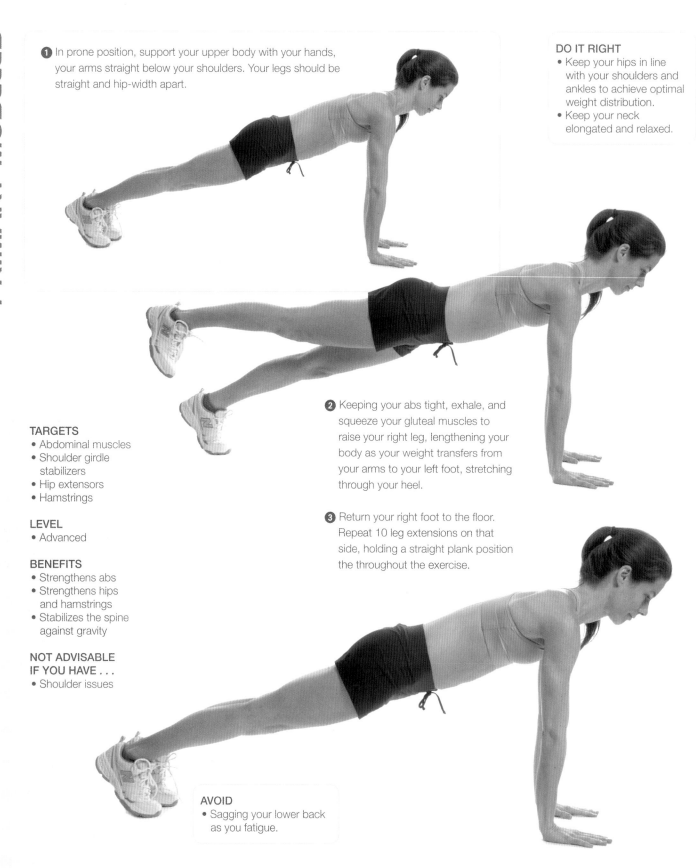

**1** In prone position, support your upper body with your hands, your arms straight below your shoulders. Your legs should be straight and hip-width apart.

### DO IT RIGHT
- Keep your hips in line with your shoulders and ankles to achieve optimal weight distribution.
- Keep your neck elongated and relaxed.

**2** Keeping your abs tight, exhale, and squeeze your gluteal muscles to raise your right leg, lengthening your body as your weight transfers from your arms to your left foot, stretching through your heel.

**3** Return your right foot to the floor. Repeat 10 leg extensions on that side, holding a straight plank position the throughout the exercise.

### TARGETS
- Abdominal muscles
- Shoulder girdle stabilizers
- Hip extensors
- Hamstrings

### LEVEL
- Advanced

### BENEFITS
- Strengthens abs
- Strengthens hips and hamstrings
- Stabilizes the spine against gravity

### NOT ADVISABLE IF YOU HAVE . . .
- Shoulder issues

### AVOID
- Sagging your lower back as you fatigue.

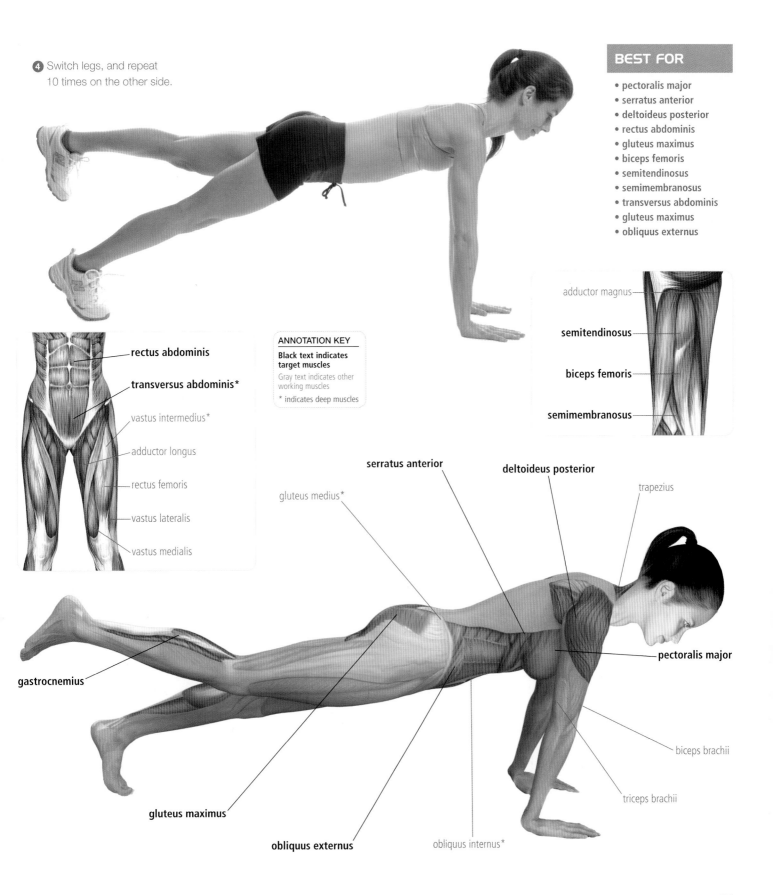

**4** Switch legs, and repeat 10 times on the other side.

**BEST FOR**

- pectoralis major
- serratus anterior
- deltoideus posterior
- rectus abdominis
- gluteus maximus
- biceps femoris
- semitendinosus
- semimembranosus
- transversus abdominis
- gluteus maximus
- obliquus externus

adductor magnus

**semitendinosus**

**biceps femoris**

**semimembranosus**

**rectus abdominis**

**transversus abdominis***

vastus intermedius*

adductor longus

rectus femoris

vastus lateralis

vastus medialis

**ANNOTATION KEY**

**Black text indicates target muscles**
Gray text indicates other working muscles
* indicates deep muscles

**serratus anterior**

gluteus medius*

**deltoideus posterior**

trapezius

**pectoralis major**

biceps brachii

triceps brachii

gastrocnemius

**gluteus maximus**

**obliquus externus**

obliquus internus*

# LOW LUNGE

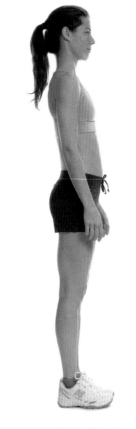

**①** Stand with your feet together and your arms hanging at your sides.

**②** Exhale, and carefully step back with your right leg, keeping it in line with your hips as you step back. The ball of your left foot should be in contact with the floor as you do the motion.

**③** Slowly slide your right foot farther back while bending your left knee, stacking it directly above your ankle.

**④** Position your palms or fingers on the floor on either side of your left leg, and slowly press your palms or fingers against the floor to enhance the placement of your upper body and your head.

**⑤** Lift your head and gaze straight forward while leaning your upper body forward and carefully rolling your shoulders down and backward.

**⑥** Press the ball of your right foot gradually into the floor, contract your thigh muscles, and press up to keep your left leg straight.

**⑦** Hold for 5 seconds. Slowly return to the starting position, and then repeat on the other side.

**AVOID**
• Dropping your back knee to the floor.

**TARGETS**
• Quadriceps
• Hamstrings
• Calf muscles

**LEVEL**
• Beginner

**BENEFITS**
• Strengthens legs and arms
• Stretches groins

**NOT ADVISABLE IF YOU HAVE . . .**
• Arm injury
• Shoulder injury
• Hip injury
• High or low blood pressure

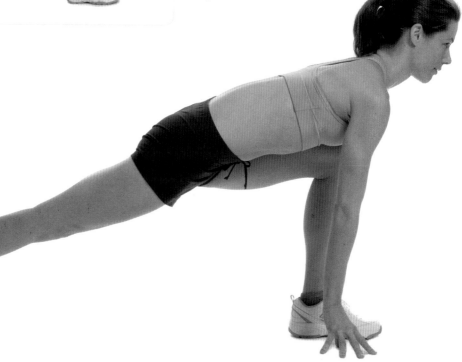

**DO IT RIGHT**
• Maintain proper position of your shoulders and your whole upper body to lengthen your spine.

**ANNOTATION KEY**
**Black text indicates target muscles**
Gray text indicates other working muscles
* indicates deep muscles

**BEST FOR**
• biceps femoris
• adductor longus
• adductor magnus
• gastrocnemius
• tibialis posterior
• iliopsoas
• rectus femoris

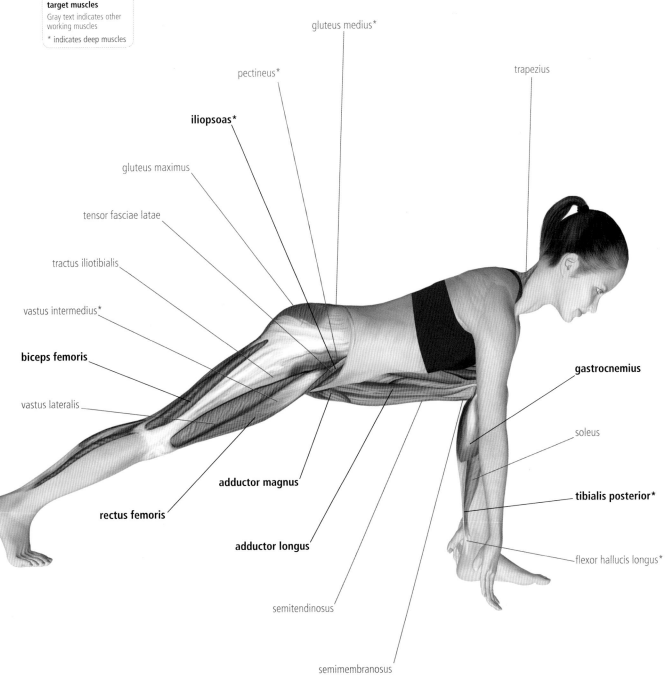

gluteus medius*

pectineus*

trapezius

**iliopsoas***

gluteus maximus

tensor fasciae latae

tractus iliotibialis

vastus intermedius*

**biceps femoris**

vastus lateralis

**gastrocnemius**

soleus

**adductor magnus**

**rectus femoris**

**tibialis posterior***

**adductor longus**

flexor hallucis longus*

semitendinosus

semimembranosus

# RESISTANCE BAND LUNGE

**1** Position a resistance band beneath one foot, grasping both handles.

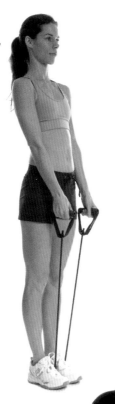

**2** Keeping your head up and your spine neutral, take a big step forward.

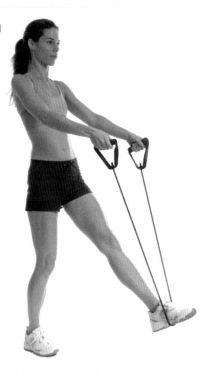

**TARGETS**
- Gluteal area
- Quadriceps

**LEVEL**
- Intermediate

**BENEFITS**
- Strengthens and tones glutes and thighs

**AVOID IF YOU HAVE . . .**
- Knee injury
- Shoulder issues

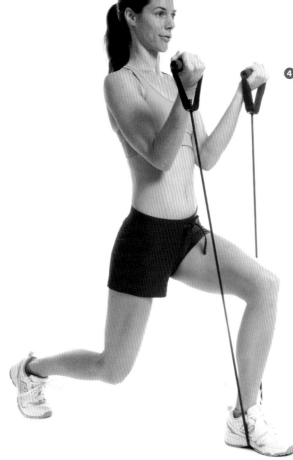

**3** Drop your back knee toward the floor, bending both legs until your front thigh is parallel to the ground. At the same time, bring the resistance band closer to your body with palms facing your shoulders.

**4** Slowly and with control, straighten your legs as you raise your body, and return your arms to starting position. Complete 15 repetitions, switch sides, and repeat for three sets of 15 on each leg.

**DO IT RIGHT**
- Keep your back straight and torso upright.
- Gaze forward.

**AVOID**
- Arching your back or allow it to curl forward.
- Twisting your torso.
- Letting your back knee touch the floor.
- Hunching your shoulders.

**BEST FOR**

- gluteus maximus
- rectus femoris
- vastus lateralis
- vastus intermedius
- vastus medialis

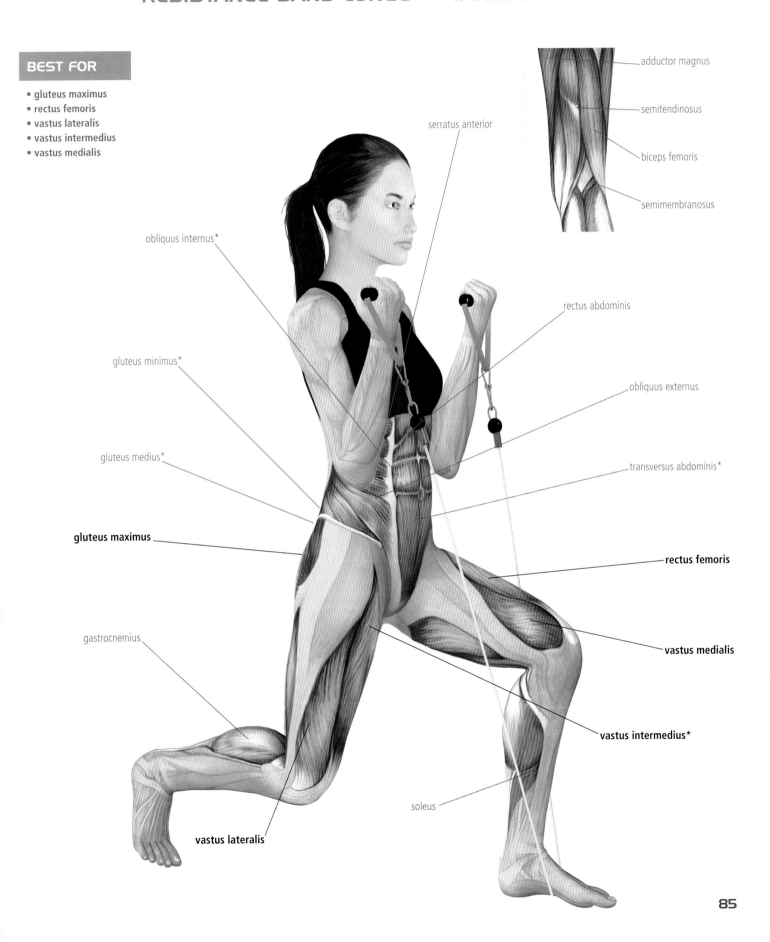

adductor magnus

semitendinosus

biceps femoris

semimembranosus

serratus anterior

obliquus internus*

rectus abdominis

gluteus minimus*

obliquus externus

gluteus medius*

transversus abdominis*

gluteus maximus

rectus femoris

vastus medialis

gastrocnemius

vastus intermedius*

soleus

vastus lateralis

# DUMBBELL LUNGE

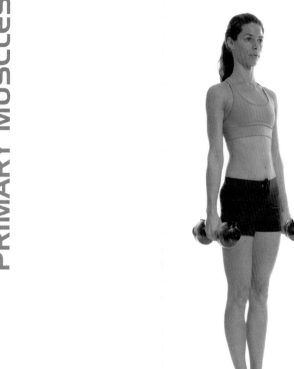

**① Stand** with your feet planted about shoulder-width apart, with your arms at your sides and a hand weight or dumbbell in each hand.

## DO IT RIGHT
- Keep your body facing forward as you step one leg in front of you.
- Stand upright.
- Gaze forward.
- Ease into the lunge.
- Make sure that your front knee is facing forward.

## TARGETS
- Gluteal area
- Quadriceps

## LEVEL
- Intermediate

## BENEFITS
- Strengthens and tones quadriceps and glutes

## NOT ADVISABLE IF YOU HAVE . . .
- Knee issues

**② Keeping** your head up and your spine neutral, take a big step forward.

**③ In one movement** as you step forward, bend your front knee to a 90-degree angle, and drop your front thigh until it is parallel to the floor. Your back knee will drop behind you so that you are balancing on the toe of your back foot, creating a straight line from your spine to the back of your knee.

**④ Push** through your front heel to stand upright, and then return to starting position. Repeat on the other leg, alternating to perform three sets of 15 lunges per leg.

## AVOID
- Turning your body to one side.
- Allowing your knee to extend past your foot.
- Arching your back.

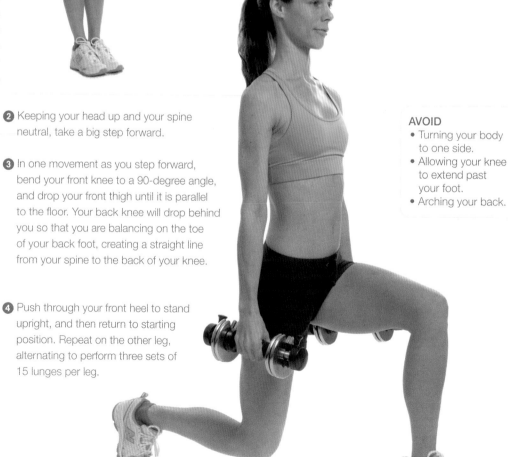

**BEST FOR**

- gluteus maximus
- rectus femoris
- vastus lateralis
- vastus intermedius
- vastus medialis

**ANNOTATION KEY**

**Black text indicates target muscles**

Gray text indicates other working muscles

* indicates deep muscles

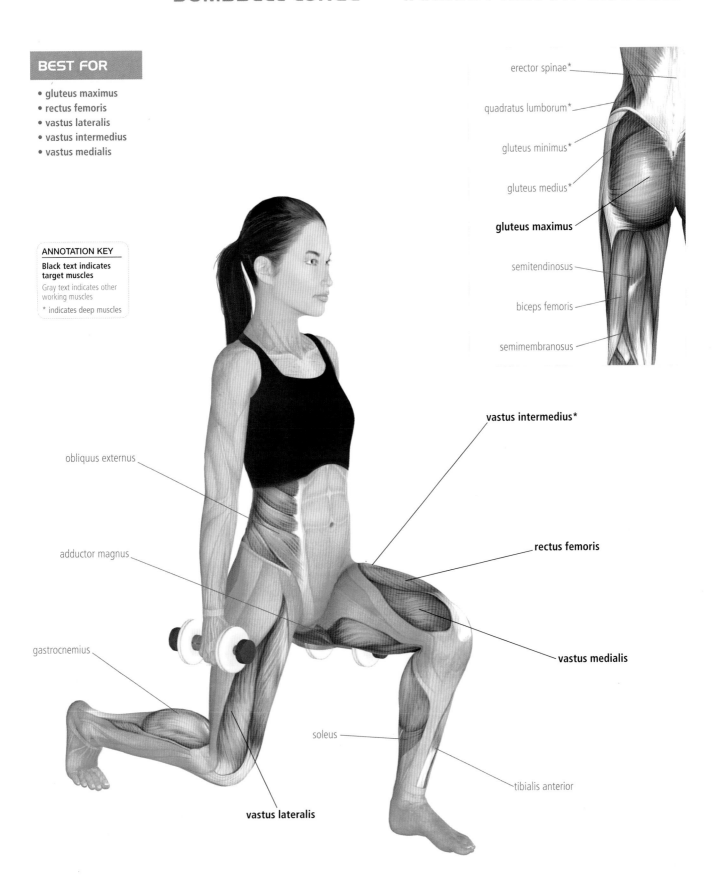

erector spinae*

quadratus lumborum*

gluteus minimus*

gluteus medius*

**gluteus maximus**

semitendinosus

biceps femoris

semimembranosus

obliquus externus

adductor magnus

gastrocnemius

**vastus intermedius***

**rectus femoris**

**vastus medialis**

soleus

tibialis anterior

**vastus lateralis**

# KNEE EXTENSION WITH ROTATION

**1** Sit upright on a chair, with your feet planted on the floor, your hands on your knees, and your gaze forward.

**2** Slowly extend and raise one leg as high as you can, or until it is parallel to the floor, with your foot flexed. Rotate it outward, pausing at the top of the circle, and then rotate your foot inward.

**3** Lower your foot, and repeat on the other side. Continue to alternate, performing two sets of 10 per side

**TARGETS**
• Inner and outer thighs

**LEVEL**
• Beginner

**BENEFITS**
• Strengthens the lateral muscles of the thigh during external rotation phase of exercise
• Strengthens the medial muscles of the thigh during internal rotation phase of exercise

**NOT ADVISABLE IF YOU HAVE . . .**
• Knee pain
• Ankle pain

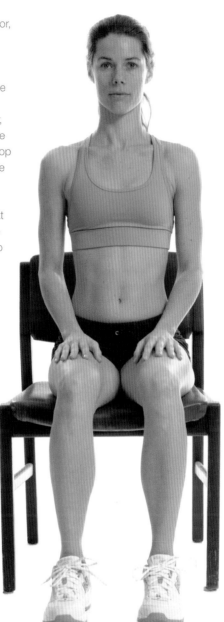

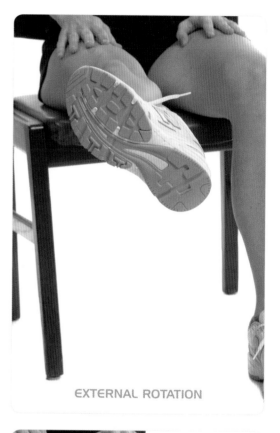

EXTERNAL ROTATION

INTERNAL ROTATION

# KNEE EXTENSION WITH ROTATION • TARGET: PRIMARY MUSCLES

## MODIFICATION

**Harder:** Wrap one end of an resistance band loop around a chair leg, the other around your ankle, and then follow steps 2 and 3.

## DO IT RIGHT
• Keep the thigh of the moving leg stabilized on the chair.

## AVOID
• Lifting your knee.

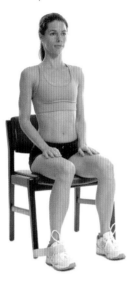

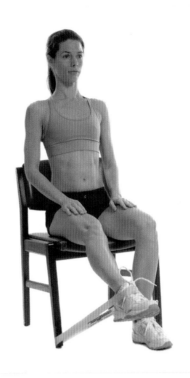

### BEST FOR

**vastus lateralis**
**vastus medialis**

---

**ANNOTATION KEY**

**Black text indicates target muscles**

Gray text indicates other working muscles

* indicates deep muscles

---

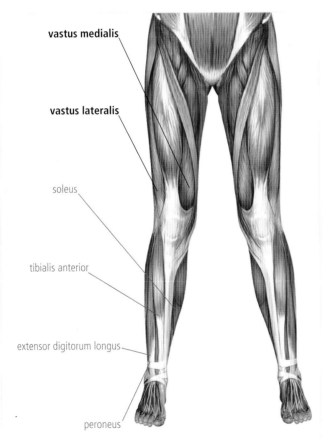

vastus medialis

vastus lateralis

soleus

tibialis anterior

extensor digitorum longus

peroneus

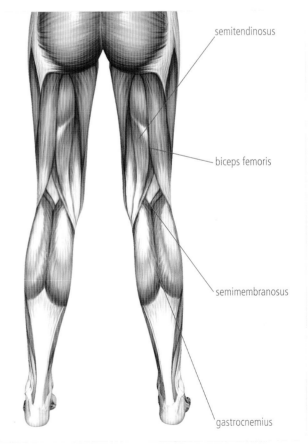

semitendinosus

biceps femoris

semimembranosus

gastrocnemius

# WALL SIT

**1** Stand with your back to a wall. Lean against the wall, and walk your feet out from under your body until your lower back rests comfortably against it.

**AVOID**
- Sitting below 90 degrees.
- Pushing your back into the wall to hold yourself up.
- Shifting from side to side as you begin to fatigue.

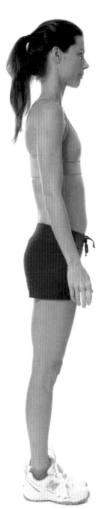

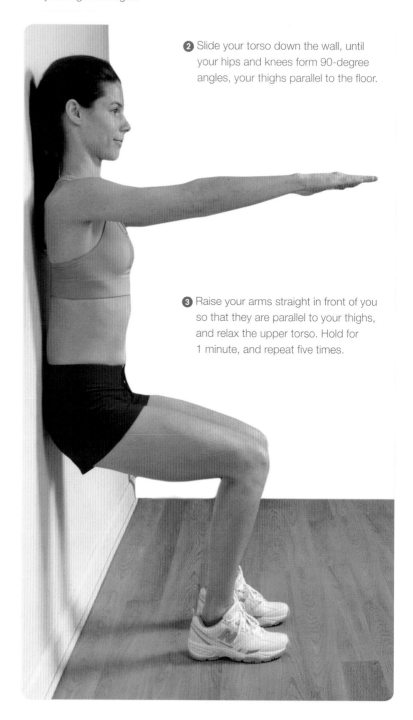

**2** Slide your torso down the wall, until your hips and knees form 90-degree angles, your thighs parallel to the floor.

**3** Raise your arms straight in front of you so that they are parallel to your thighs, and relax the upper torso. Hold for 1 minute, and repeat five times.

**TARGETS**
- Quadriceps
- Gluteal area

**LEVEL**
- Intermediate

**BENEFITS**
- Strengthens quadriceps and gluteal muscles
- Trains the body to place weight evenly between the legs

**NOT ADVISABLE IF YOU HAVE . . .**
- Knee pain

**DO IT RIGHT**
- Keep your body firm throughout the exercise.
- Relax your shoulders and neck.
- Form a 90-degree angle with your hips and knees to receive maximum benefit from the exercise.

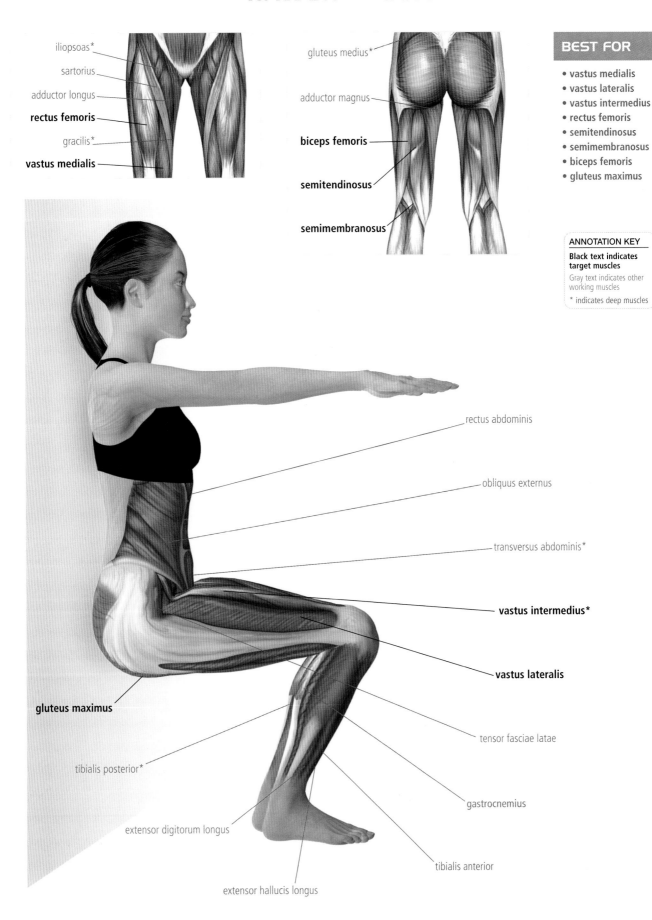

iliopsoas*
sartorius
adductor longus
**rectus femoris**
gracilis*
**vastus medialis**

gluteus medius*
adductor magnus
**biceps femoris**
**semitendinosus**
**semimembranosus**

**BEST FOR**

- vastus medialis
- vastus lateralis
- vastus intermedius
- rectus femoris
- semitendinosus
- semimembranosus
- biceps femoris
- gluteus maximus

**ANNOTATION KEY**

**Black text indicates target muscles**
Gray text indicates other working muscles
* indicates deep muscles

rectus abdominis
obliquus externus
transversus abdominis*
**vastus intermedius***
**vastus lateralis**
tensor fasciae latae
gastrocnemius
tibialis anterior

**gluteus maximus**
tibialis posterior*
extensor digitorum longus
extensor hallucis longus

# SWISS BALL WALL SIT

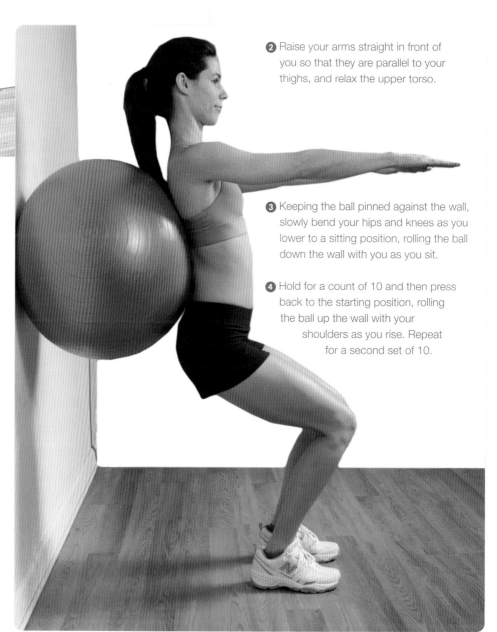

**1** Place a Swiss ball against a wall and stand with your back to it so that your back and shoulders are pinning it to the wall. Your feet should be about hip-width apart, but slightly ahead of your hips.

**AVOID**
- Sitting below 90 degrees.
- Shifting from side to side as you begin to fatigue.

**DO IT RIGHT**
- Place your feet ahead of your hips by half the length of your thigh.
- Keep your body firm throughout the exercise.
- Relax your shoulders and neck.

**2** Raise your arms straight in front of you so that they are parallel to your thighs, and relax the upper torso.

**3** Keeping the ball pinned against the wall, slowly bend your hips and knees as you lower to a sitting position, rolling the ball down the wall with you as you sit.

**4** Hold for a count of 10 and then press back to the starting position, rolling the ball up the wall with your shoulders as you rise. Repeat for a second set of 10.

**TARGETS**
- Quadriceps
- Gluteal area

**LEVEL**
- Intermediate

**BENEFITS**
- Strengthens quadriceps and gluteal muscles
- Trains the body to place weight evenly between the legs

**NOT ADVISABLE IF YOU HAVE . . .**
- Knee pain

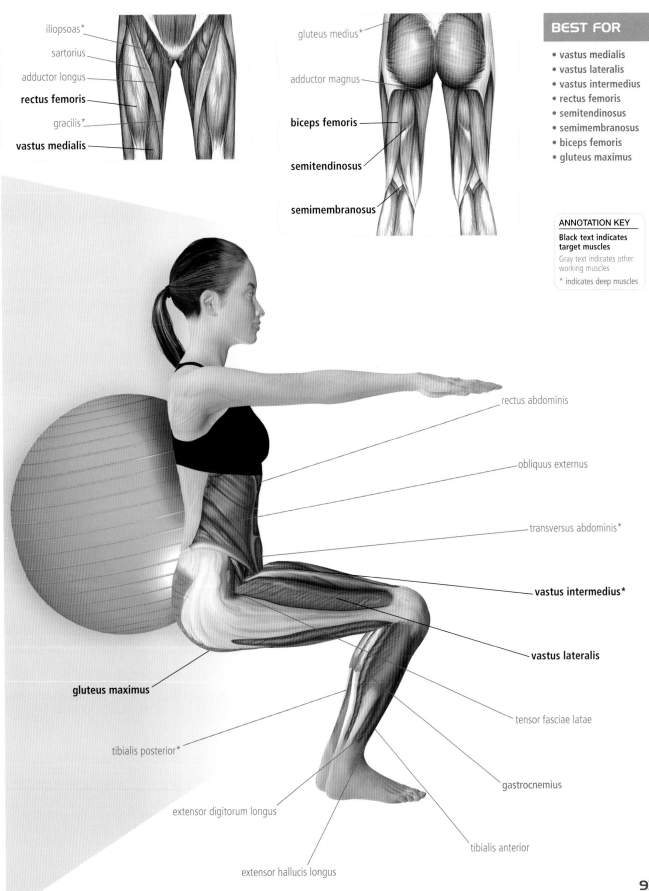

iliopsoas*
sartorius
adductor longus
**rectus femoris**
gracilis*
**vastus medialis**

gluteus medius*
adductor magnus
**biceps femoris**
**semitendinosus**
**semimembranosus**

**BEST FOR**

- vastus medialis
- vastus lateralis
- vastus intermedius
- rectus femoris
- semitendinosus
- semimembranosus
- biceps femoris
- gluteus maximus

**ANNOTATION KEY**

**Black text indicates target muscles**
Gray text indicates other working muscles
* indicates deep muscles

rectus abdominis

obliquus externus

transversus abdominis*

**vastus intermedius***

**vastus lateralis**

tensor fasciae latae

gastrocnemius

**gluteus maximus**

tibialis posterior*

extensor digitorum longus

extensor hallucis longus

tibialis anterior

93

# LATERAL LOW LUNGE

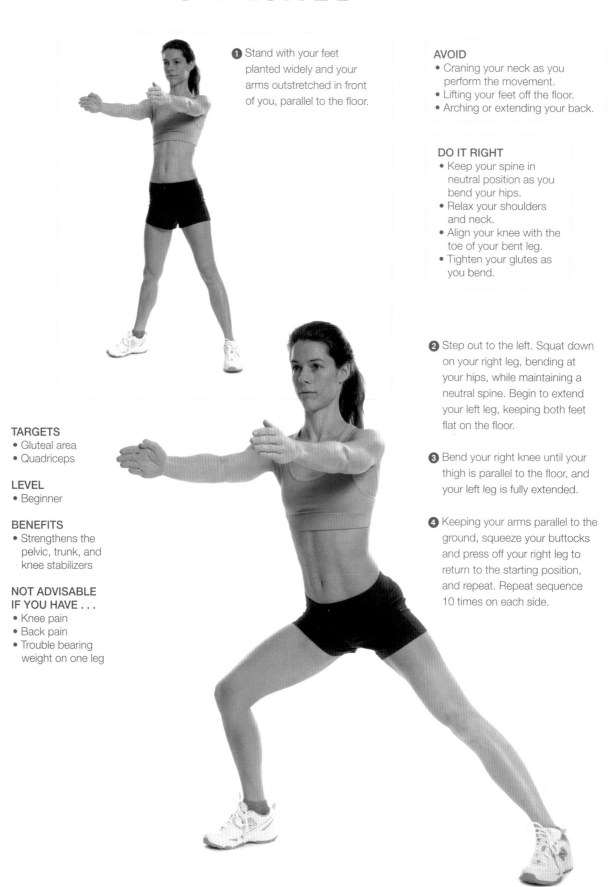

**1** Stand with your feet planted widely and your arms outstretched in front of you, parallel to the floor.

**AVOID**
- Craning your neck as you perform the movement.
- Lifting your feet off the floor.
- Arching or extending your back.

**DO IT RIGHT**
- Keep your spine in neutral position as you bend your hips.
- Relax your shoulders and neck.
- Align your knee with the toe of your bent leg.
- Tighten your glutes as you bend.

**2** Step out to the left. Squat down on your right leg, bending at your hips, while maintaining a neutral spine. Begin to extend your left leg, keeping both feet flat on the floor.

**3** Bend your right knee until your thigh is parallel to the floor, and your left leg is fully extended.

**4** Keeping your arms parallel to the ground, squeeze your buttocks and press off your right leg to return to the starting position, and repeat. Repeat sequence 10 times on each side.

**TARGETS**
- Gluteal area
- Quadriceps

**LEVEL**
- Beginner

**BENEFITS**
- Strengthens the pelvic, trunk, and knee stabilizers

**NOT ADVISABLE IF YOU HAVE . . .**
- Knee pain
- Back pain
- Trouble bearing weight on one leg

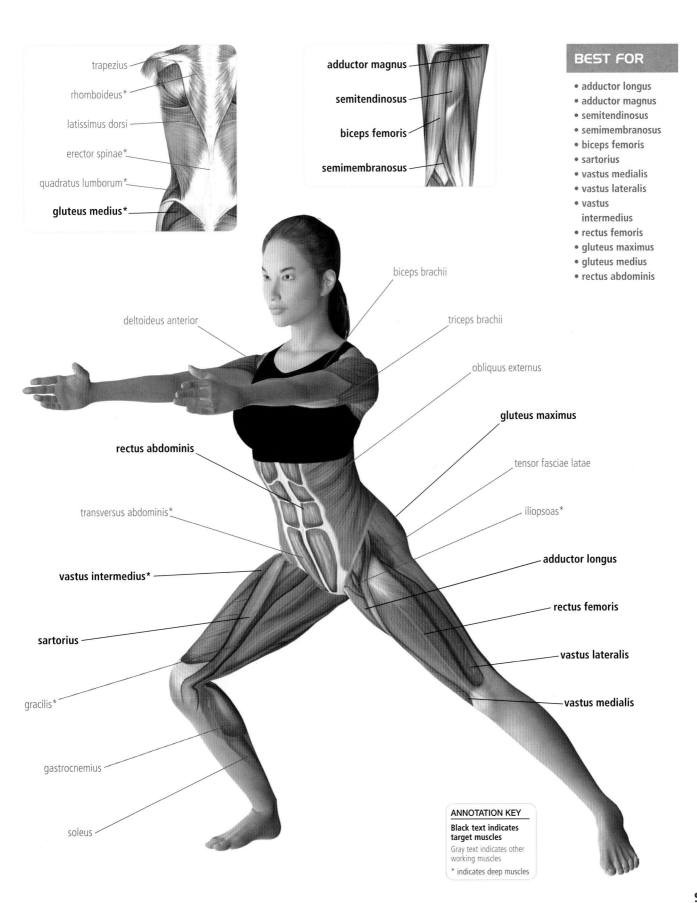

trapezius

rhomboideus*

latissimus dorsi

erector spinae*

quadratus lumborum*

**gluteus medius***

**adductor magnus**

**semitendinosus**

**biceps femoris**

**semimembranosus**

biceps brachii

deltoideus anterior

triceps brachii

obliquus externus

**gluteus maximus**

**rectus abdominis**

tensor fasciae latae

iliopsoas*

transversus abdominis*

**adductor longus**

**vastus intermedius***

**rectus femoris**

**sartorius**

**vastus lateralis**

gracilis*

**vastus medialis**

gastrocnemius

soleus

**ANNOTATION KEY**

**Black text indicates target muscles**

Gray text indicates other working muscles

* indicates deep muscles

# STEP-DOWN

**1** Standing up straight on a firm step or block, plant your left foot firmly close to the edge, and allow the right foot to hang off the side. Flex the toes of your right foot.

**DO IT RIGHT**
- Align your bent knee with your second toe so that your knee doesn't rotate inward.
- Bend your knees and hips at the same time.
- Keep your hips behind your foot, leaning your torso forward as you lower into the bend.

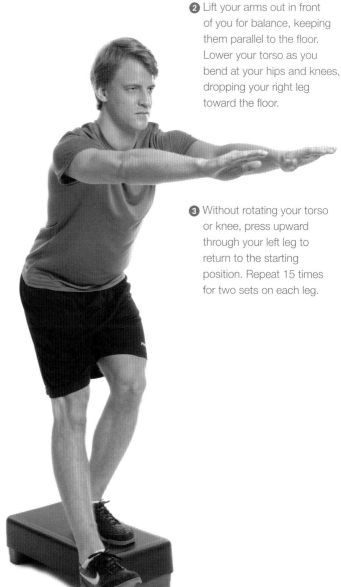

**2** Lift your arms out in front of you for balance, keeping them parallel to the floor. Lower your torso as you bend at your hips and knees, dropping your right leg toward the floor.

**3** Without rotating your torso or knee, press upward through your left leg to return to the starting position. Repeat 15 times for two sets on each leg.

**TARGETS**
- Quadriceps
- Gluteal area

**LEVEL**
- Beginner

**BENEFITS**
- Strengthens pelvic and knee stabilizers

**NOT ADVISABLE IF YOU HAVE . . .**
- Ankle pain
- Sharp knee pain
- Lower-back pain

**AVOID**
- Craning your neck.
- Placing weight on the foot being lowered to the floor—only allow a touch.

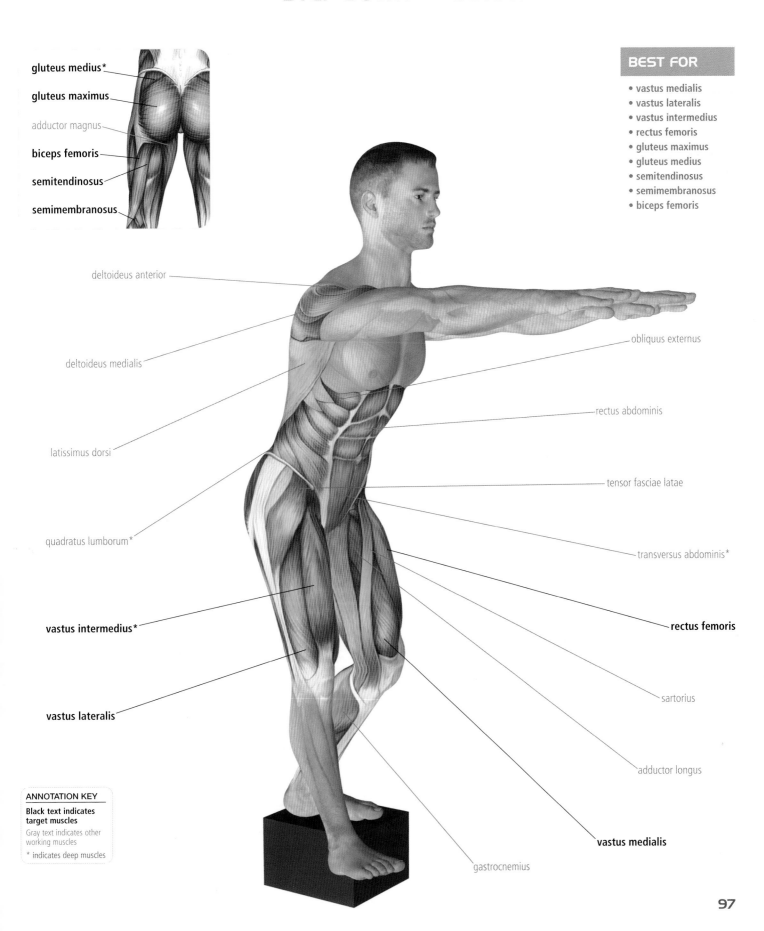

gluteus medius*

gluteus maximus

adductor magnus

biceps femoris

semitendinosus

semimembranosus

**BEST FOR**

• vastus medialis
• vastus lateralis
• vastus intermedius
• rectus femoris
• gluteus maximus
• gluteus medius
• semitendinosus
• semimembranosus
• biceps femoris

deltoideus anterior

deltoideus medialis

latissimus dorsi

quadratus lumborum*

vastus intermedius*

vastus lateralis

obliquus externus

rectus abdominis

tensor fasciae latae

transversus abdominis*

**rectus femoris**

sartorius

adductor longus

**vastus medialis**

gastrocnemius

**ANNOTATION KEY**

**Black text indicates target muscles**

Gray text indicates other working muscles

* indicates deep muscles

# POWER SQUAT

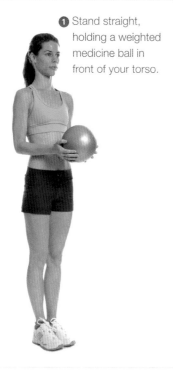

**1** Stand straight, holding a weighted medicine ball in front of your torso.

**2** Shift your weight to your left foot, and bend your right knee, lifting your right foot toward your buttocks. Bend your elbows and draw the ball toward the outside of your right ear.

### DO IT RIGHT
- Move the ball in an arc through the air.
- Keep your hips and knees aligned throughout the movement.
- Relax your neck and shoulders.

### TARGETS
- Abdominals
- Hip flexors

### LEVEL
- Advanced

### BENEFITS
- Improves balance
- Stabilizes pelvis, trunk, and knees
- Promotes stronger movement patterns

### NOT ADVISABLE IF YOU HAVE . . .
- Knee pain
- Lower-back pain
- Shoulder pain

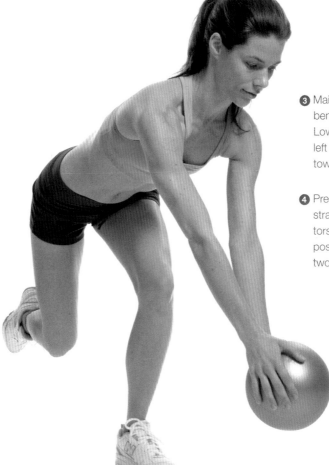

**3** Maintaining a neutral spine, bend at your hips and knee. Lower your torso toward your left side, bringing the ball toward your left ankle.

**4** Press into your left leg and straighten your knee and torso, returning to the starting position. Repeat 15 times for two sets on each leg.

### AVOID
- Allowing your knee to extend beyond your toes as you bend and rotate.
- Moving your foot from its starting position.
- Flexing your spine.

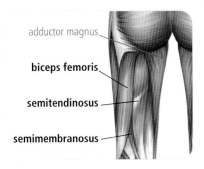

adductor magnus

**biceps femoris**

**semitendinosus**

**semimembranosus**

## BEST FOR

- semitendinosus
- semimembranosus
- biceps femoris
- vastus medialis
- vastus lateralis
- rectus femoris

- gluteus maximus
- gluteus medius
- piriformis
- erector spinae
- tibialis anterior
- tibialis posterior

- soleus
- gastrocnemius
- deltoideus medialis
- infraspinatus
- supraspinatus
- teres minor

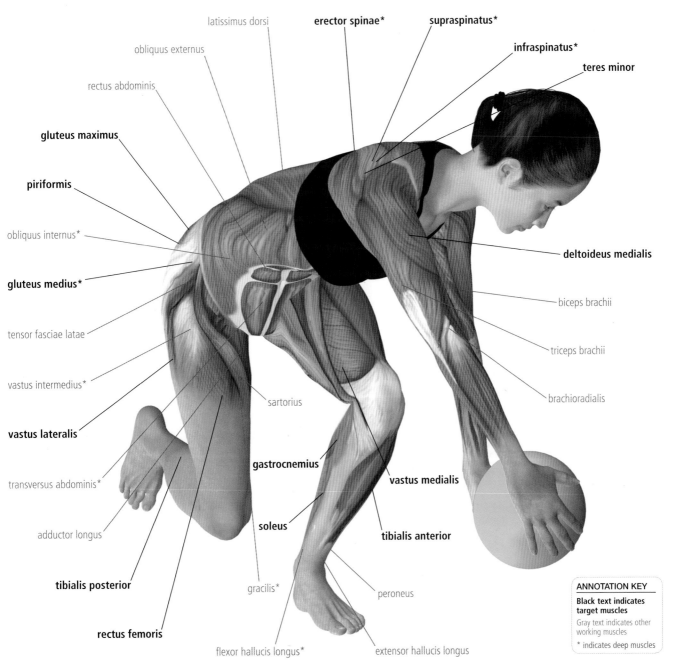

latissimus dorsi

obliquus externus

rectus abdominis

**gluteus maximus**

**piriformis**

obliquus internus*

**gluteus medius***

tensor fasciae latae

vastus intermedius*

**vastus lateralis**

transversus abdominis*

adductor longus

**tibialis posterior**

**rectus femoris**

flexor hallucis longus*

gracilis*

**erector spinae***

**supraspinatus***

**infraspinatus***

teres minor

**deltoideus medialis**

biceps brachii

triceps brachii

brachioradialis

sartorius

**gastrocnemius**

**vastus medialis**

**soleus**

**tibialis anterior**

peroneus

extensor hallucis longus

### ANNOTATION KEY

**Black text indicates target muscles**

Gray text indicates other working muscles

* indicates deep muscles

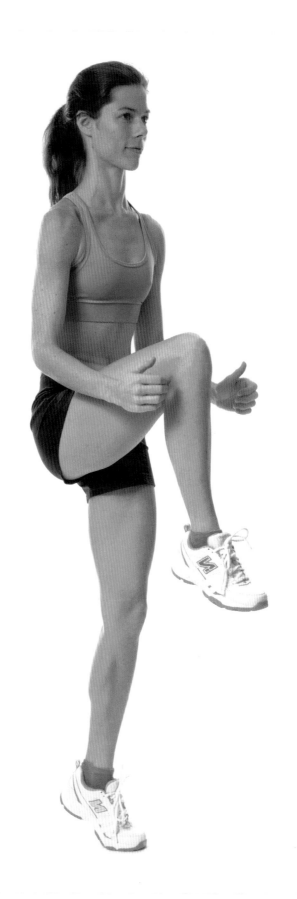

# TARGET: SECONDARY MUSCLES

Running demands that your entire body works hard, including your core, back, shoulders, and arms. Building strength in these secondary areas will help you run more efficiently, with greater endurance and a lowered risk of injury.

Your core is made up of the deep muscle layers that lie close to the spine, including the abdominals (rectus abdominis, transversus abdominis, obliquus externus, and obliquus internus), the spinal extensors (multifidus spinae, erector spinae, splenius, and semispinalis), and the diaphragm. During a run, it stabilizes your trunk and pelvis, allowing the arms and legs to move properly. Working on the minor core muscles, such as the latissimus dorsi (the large smooth muscle of your back) and the trapezius (the triangle-shaped muscle on the upper back and neck), will also help you run better and strengthen your back. When devising your exercise plan, don't forget the arms and shoulders, which must pump effectively to keep you balanced as you move. Included here are exercises that target these muscles, too, including the deltoids, biceps, and triceps.

# UNILATERAL LEG CIRCLES

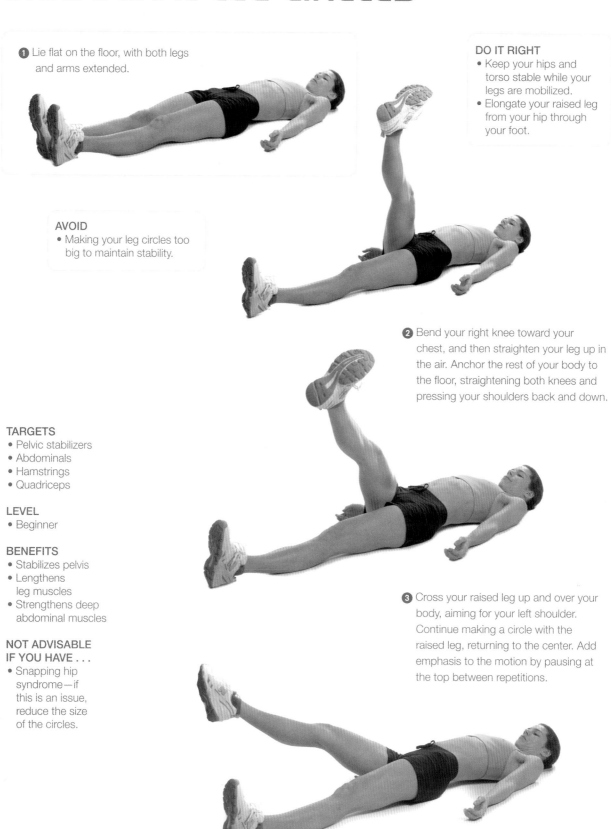

**1** Lie flat on the floor, with both legs and arms extended.

**DO IT RIGHT**
• Keep your hips and torso stable while your legs are mobilized.
• Elongate your raised leg from your hip through your foot.

**AVOID**
• Making your leg circles too big to maintain stability.

**2** Bend your right knee toward your chest, and then straighten your leg up in the air. Anchor the rest of your body to the floor, straightening both knees and pressing your shoulders back and down.

**TARGETS**
• Pelvic stabilizers
• Abdominals
• Hamstrings
• Quadriceps

**LEVEL**
• Beginner

**BENEFITS**
• Stabilizes pelvis
• Lengthens leg muscles
• Strengthens deep abdominal muscles

**NOT ADVISABLE IF YOU HAVE . . .**
• Snapping hip syndrome—if this is an issue, reduce the size of the circles.

**3** Cross your raised leg up and over your body, aiming for your left shoulder. Continue making a circle with the raised leg, returning to the center. Add emphasis to the motion by pausing at the top between repetitions.

**4** Switch directions so that you aim your leg away from your body. Repeat with the other leg. Complete full movement five to eight times.

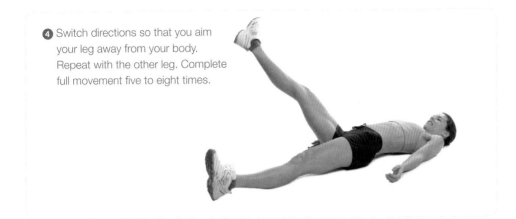

**BEST FOR**

- rectus abdominis
- obliquus externus
- rectus femoris
- biceps femoris
- triceps brachii
- gluteus maximus
- adductor magnus
- vastus lateralis
- vastus medialis
- tensor fasciae latae

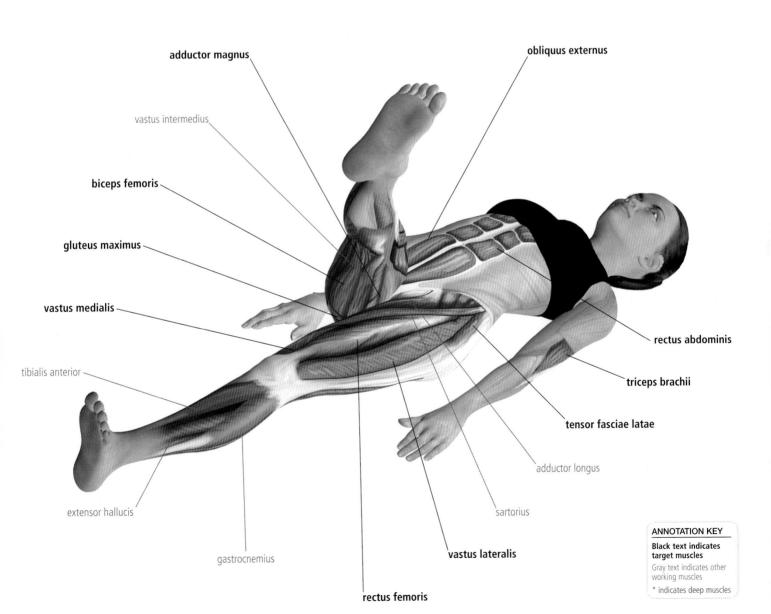

adductor magnus

vastus intermedius

biceps femoris

gluteus maximus

vastus medialis

tibialis anterior

extensor hallucis

gastrocnemius

rectus femoris

obliquus externus

rectus abdominis

triceps brachii

tensor fasciae latae

adductor longus

sartorius

vastus lateralis

**ANNOTATION KEY**

**Black text indicates target muscles**

Gray text indicates other working muscles

* indicates deep muscles

# QUADRUPED LEG LIFT

**1** Kneeling on all fours, connect with your abdominals by drawing your navel up toward your spine.

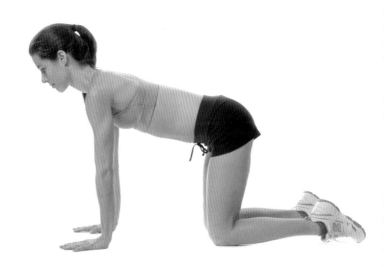

**DO IT RIGHT**
- Keep your movement slow and steady to decrease pelvic rotation.
- Engage your abs by drawing your navel toward your spine.
- Press your shoulder blades down and back.

**2** Slowly raise your right arm and extend your left leg, all while keeping your torso still. Extend your arm and leg until they are both parallel to the floor, creating one long line with your body. Do not allow your pelvis to bend or rotate.

**3** Bring your arm and leg back into the starting position.

**TARGETS**
- Abdominals
- Pelvic stabilizers
- Hip extensors
- Obliques

**LEVEL**
- Beginner

**BENEFITS**
- Tones arms, legs, and abdominals

**NOT ADVISABLE IF YOU HAVE . . .**
- Wrist pain
- Lower-back pain
- Knee pain while kneeling
- Inability to stabilize the spine while moving limbs

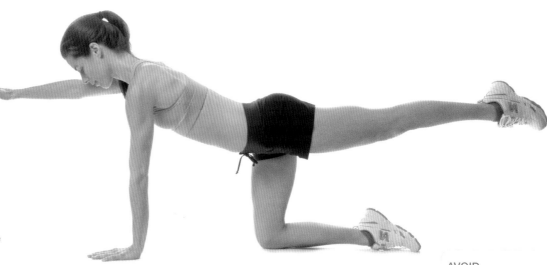

**4** Repeat sequence on the other side, alternating sides six times.

**AVOID**
- Tilting your pelvis during the movement—slide your leg along the surface of the floor before lifting.
- Allowing your back to sink into an arched position.

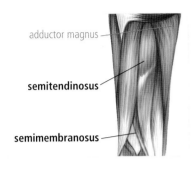

adductor magnus

**semitendinosus**

**semimembranosus**

**MODIFICATION**

**Harder:** Follow steps 1 and 2, and then draw your opposite knee and elbow inward to touch. Repeat entire sequence on the other side.

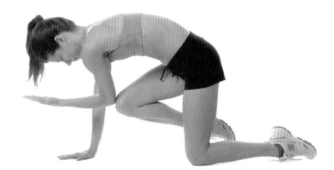

**ANNOTATION KEY**

**Black text indicates target muscles**

Gray text indicates other working muscles

* indicates deep muscles

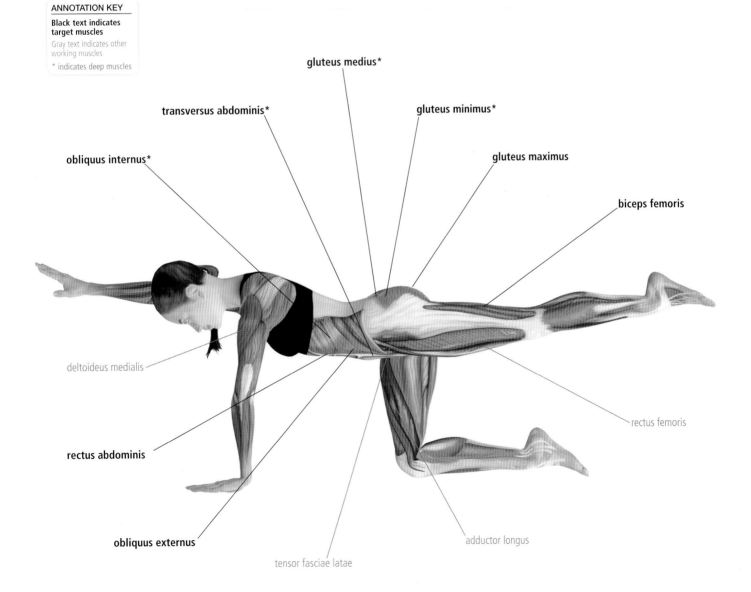

gluteus medius*

transversus abdominis*

gluteus minimus*

obliquus internus*

gluteus maximus

biceps femoris

deltoideus medialis

rectus femoris

**rectus abdominis**

**obliquus externus**

tensor fasciae latae

adductor longus

# FRONT PLANK

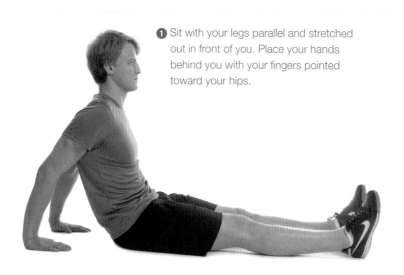

**①** Sit with your legs parallel and stretched out in front of you. Place your hands behind you with your fingers pointed toward your hips.

**DO IT RIGHT**
- Elevate your pelvis throughout the exercise.

**AVOID**
- Allowing your shoulders to sink into their sockets— if your legs do not feel strong enough to support your body, slightly bend your knees.

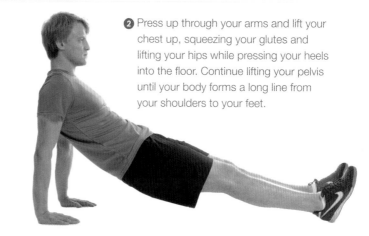

**②** Press up through your arms and lift your chest up, squeezing your glutes and lifting your hips while pressing your heels into the floor. Continue lifting your pelvis until your body forms a long line from your shoulders to your feet.

**TARGETS**
- Hip extensors
- Core stabilizers
- Shoulders
- Thighs

**LEVEL**
- Advanced

**BENEFITS**
- Strengthens core muscles and deep stabilizing muscles

**NOT ADVISABLE IF YOU HAVE . . .**
- Wrist pain
- Knee pain
- Shoulder injury
- Shooting pains down leg

**③** Without allowing your pelvis to drop, raise your left leg, straightened, in the air.

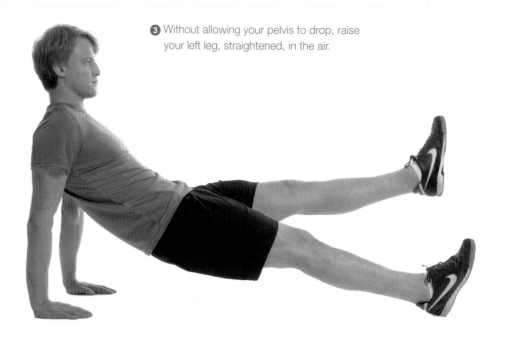

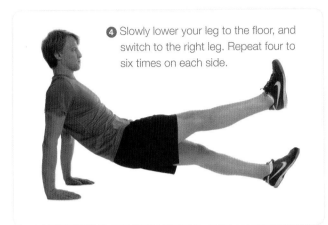

**4** Slowly lower your leg to the floor, and switch to the right leg. Repeat four to six times on each side.

## BEST FOR

- gluteus maximus
- biceps femoris
- deltoideus
- rectus femoris
- adductor magnus
- tensor fasciae latae
- rectus abdominis
- transversus abdominis
- adductor longus
- obliquus externus
- latissimus dorsi
- triceps brachii

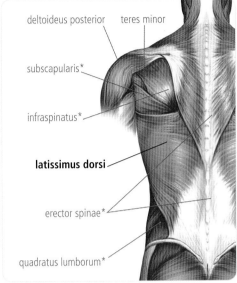

deltoideus posterior · teres minor

subscapularis*

infraspinatus*

**latissimus dorsi**

erector spinae*

quadratus lumborum*

### ANNOTATION KEY

**Black text indicates target muscles**

Gray text indicates other working muscles

\* indicates deep muscles

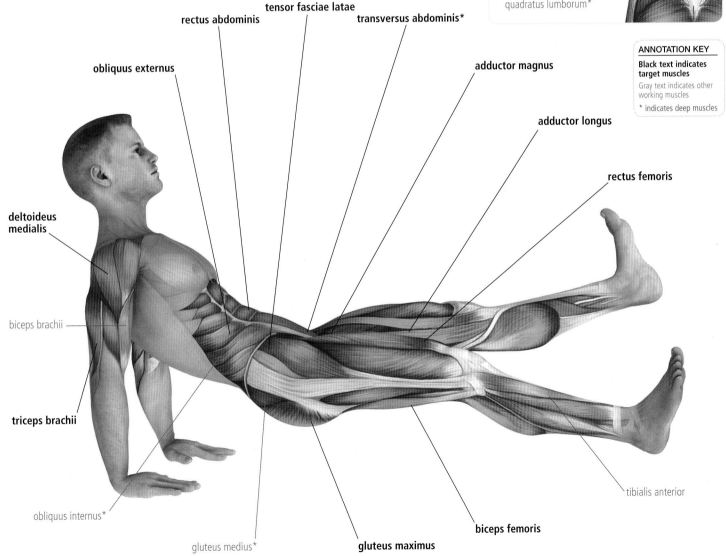

rectus abdominis

tensor fasciae latae

transversus abdominis*

obliquus externus

adductor magnus

adductor longus

rectus femoris

deltoideus medialis

biceps brachii

triceps brachii

tibialis anterior

obliquus internus*

biceps femoris

gluteus medius*

gluteus maximus

# SWIMMING

**1** Lie prone on the floor with your legs hip-width apart. Stretch your arms beside your ears on the floor. Engage your pelvic floor, and draw your navel into your spine.

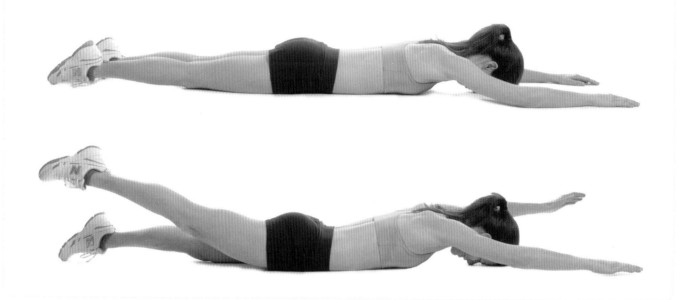

**TARGETS**
• Spinal extensors
• Hip extensors

**LEVEL**
• Beginner

**BENEFITS**
• Strengthens hip and spine extensors
• Challenges stabilization of the spine against rotation

**NOT ADVISABLE IF YOU HAVE . . .**
• Lower-back pain
• Extreme curvature of the upper spine
• Curvature of the lower spine

**2** Extend through your upper back as you lift your left arm and right leg simultaneously. Lift your head and shoulders off the floor.

**3** Lower your arm and leg to the starting position, maintaining a stretch in your limbs throughout.

**DO IT RIGHT**
• Extend your limbs as far as possible in opposite directions.
• Squeeze your glutes, and draw your navel into your spine throughout the exercise.
• Keep your neck to remain long and relaxed.

**AVOID**
• Allowing your shoulders to lift toward your ears.

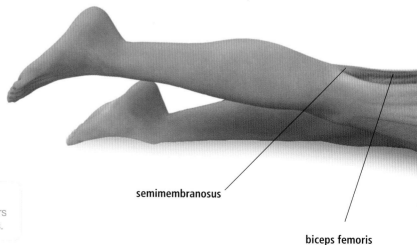

semimembranosus

biceps femoris

**4** Extend your right arm and left leg off the floor, lengthening and lifting your head and shoulders.

**5** Elongate your limbs as you return to the starting position. Repeat six to eight times.

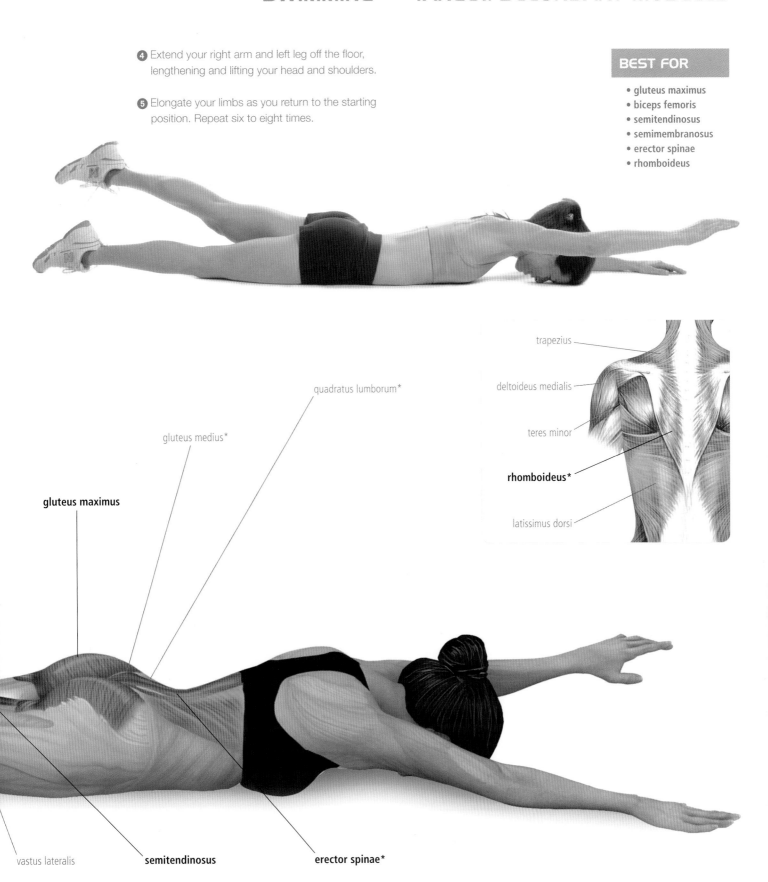

trapezius

deltoideus medialis

teres minor

**rhomboideus***

latissimus dorsi

quadratus lumborum*

gluteus medius*

**gluteus maximus**

vastus lateralis

**semitendinosus**

**erector spinae***

# BASIC CRUNCH

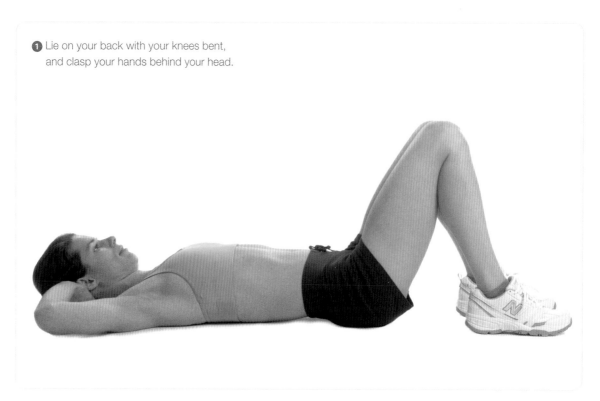

**1** Lie on your back with your knees bent, and clasp your hands behind your head.

**2** Keeping your elbows wide, engage your abdominals, and lift your upper torso to achieve a crunching movement.

**3** Slowly return to the starting position. Repeat 15 times for two sets.

**TARGETS**
• Abdominals

**LEVEL**
• Beginner

**BENEFITS**
• Strengthens the torso
• Improves pelvic and core stability

**NOT ADVISABLE IF YOU HAVE . . .**
• Back pain
• Neck pain

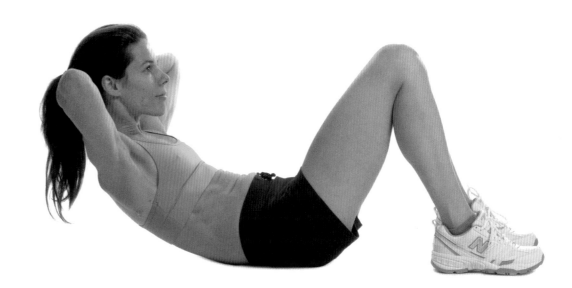

## DO IT RIGHT
- Use your shoulders and abdominals to initiate the movement.
- Keep your pelvis in neutral position during the crunching motion.
- Slightly tuck your chin, directing your gaze toward the inner thighs.

## AVOID
- Pulling from the neck.
- Tilting your hips toward the floor.

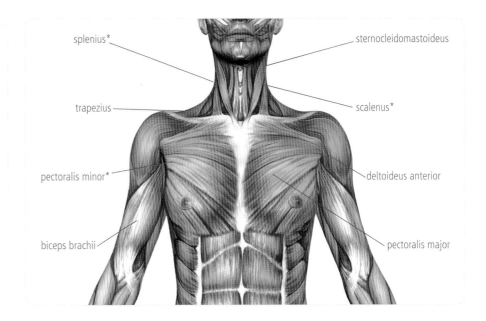

splenius*

sternocleidomastoideus

trapezius

scalenus*

pectoralis minor*

deltoideus anterior

biceps brachii

pectoralis major

## ANNOTATION KEY
**Black text indicates target muscles**

Gray text indicates other working muscles

\* indicates deep muscles

## BEST FOR
- rectus abdominis
- obliquus internus
- obliquus externus
- transversus abdominis

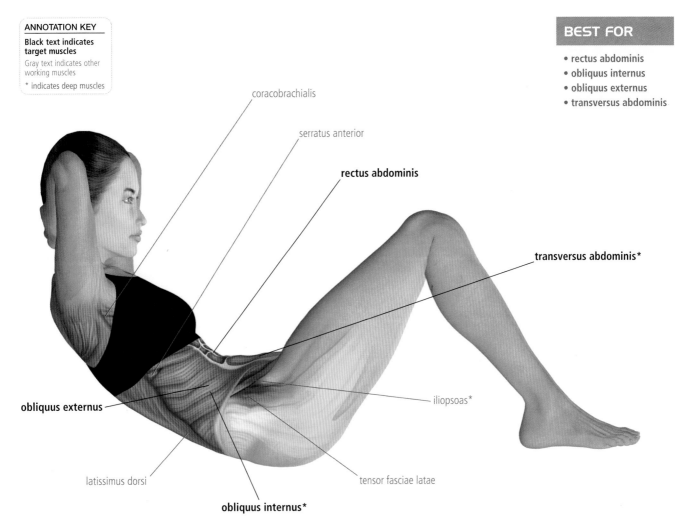

coracobrachialis

serratus anterior

**rectus abdominis**

**transversus abdominis\***

**obliquus externus**

iliopsoas*

latissimus dorsi

tensor fasciae latae

**obliquus internus\***

# CROSSOVER CRUNCH

**1** Bring your hands behind your head, and lift your legs off the floor into a tabletop position, so that your thighs and calves form a 90-degree angle.

**DO IT RIGHT**
• Elongate your neck.
• Lift your chin away from your chest.
• Keep both hips stable on the floor.

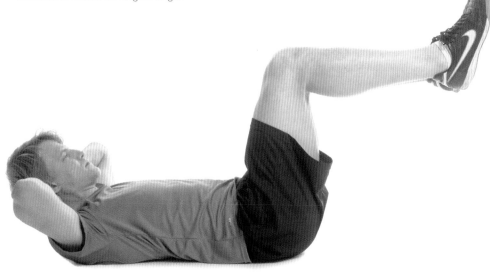

**TARGETS**
• Torso stabilizers
• Abdominals

**LEVEL**
• Intermediate

**BENEFITS**
• Stabilizes core
• Strengthens abdominals

**NOT ADVISABLE IF YOU HAVE . . .**
• Neck issues
• Lower-back pain

**2** Roll up with your torso, reaching your right elbow to your left knee and extending the right leg in front of you. Imagine pulling your shoulder blades off the floor and twisting from your ribs and oblique muscles.

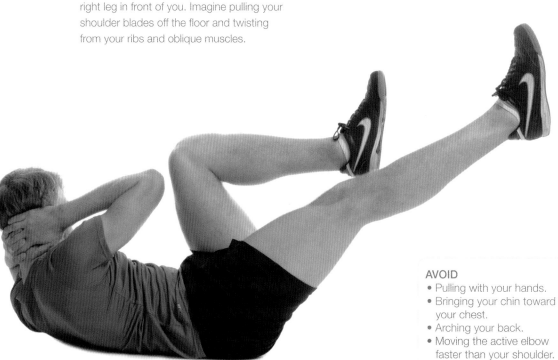

**AVOID**
• Pulling with your hands.
• Bringing your chin toward your chest.
• Arching your back.
• Moving the active elbow faster than your shoulder.

# CROSSOVER CRUNCH • TARGET: SECONDARY MUSCLES

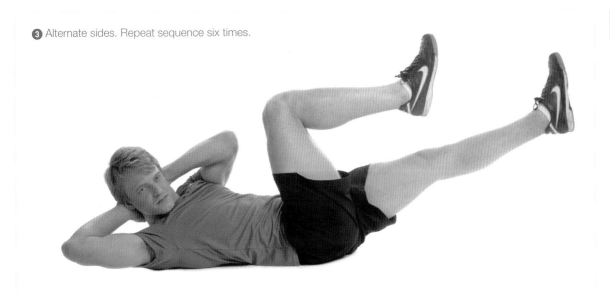

**3** Alternate sides. Repeat sequence six times.

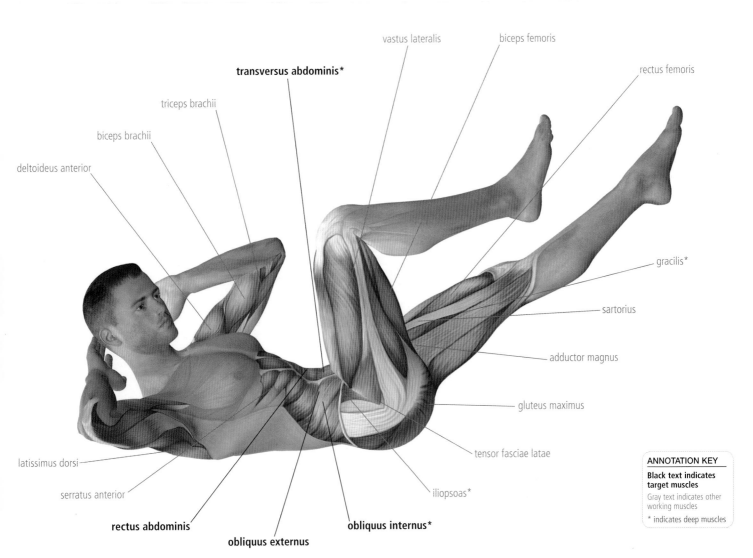

vastus lateralis

biceps femoris

rectus femoris

**transversus abdominis***

triceps brachii

biceps brachii

deltoideus anterior

gracilis*

sartorius

adductor magnus

gluteus maximus

tensor fasciae latae

latissimus dorsi

iliopsoas*

serratus anterior

**rectus abdominis**

**obliquus externus**

**obliquus internus***

### ANNOTATION KEY

**Black text indicates target muscles**

Gray text indicates other working muscles

* indicates deep muscles

# ABDOMINAL KICK

❶ Pull your right knee toward your chest and straighten your left leg, raising it about 45 degrees from the floor.

❷ Place your right hand on your right ankle, and your left hand on your right knee (this maintains proper alignment of leg).

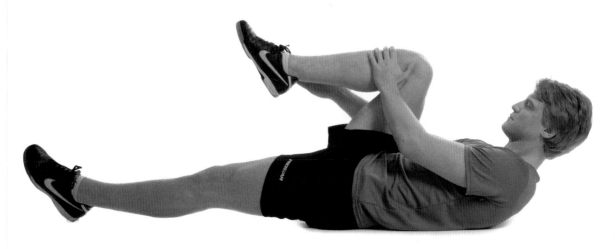

❸ Switch your legs two times, switching your hand placement simultaneously.

**TARGETS**
- Torso stabilizers
- Abdominals

**LEVEL**
- Intermediate

**BENEFITS**
- Stabilizes core while extremities are in motion
- Strengthens abdominals

**NOT ADVISABLE IF YOU HAVE . . .**
- Neck issues
- Lower-back pain

**AVOID**
- Allowing your lower back to rise up off the floor; use your abdominals to stabilize your core while switching legs.

**DO IT RIGHT**
- Place your outside hand on the ankle of your bent leg and your inside hand on your bent knee.
- Keep your chest lifted.

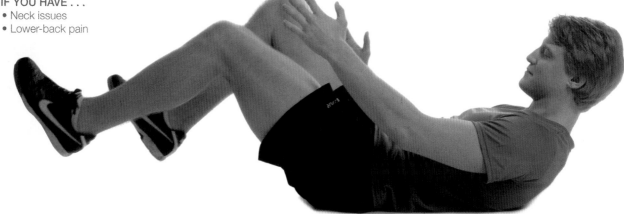

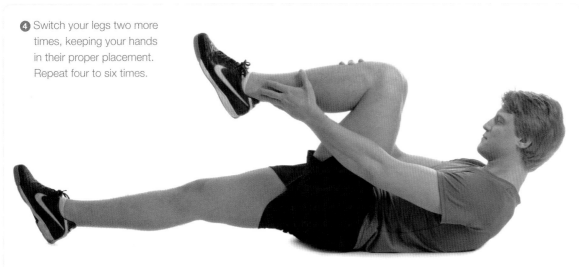

**④** Switch your legs two more times, keeping your hands in their proper placement. Repeat four to six times.

**ANNOTATION KEY**

**Black text indicates target muscles**
Gray text indicates other working muscles
* indicates deep muscles

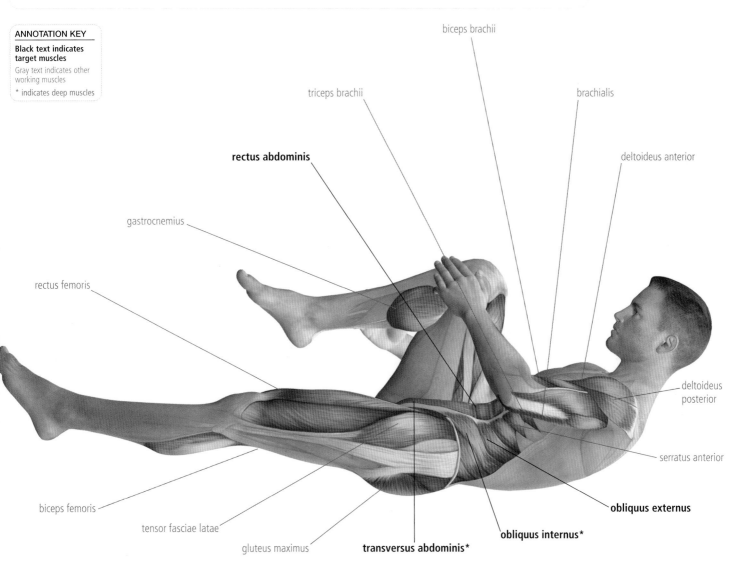

biceps brachii

triceps brachii

brachialis

**rectus abdominis**

deltoideus anterior

gastrocnemius

rectus femoris

deltoideus posterior

serratus anterior

biceps femoris

**obliquus externus**

tensor fasciae latae

**obliquus internus***

gluteus maximus

**transversus abdominis***

# PLANK KNEE PULL-IN

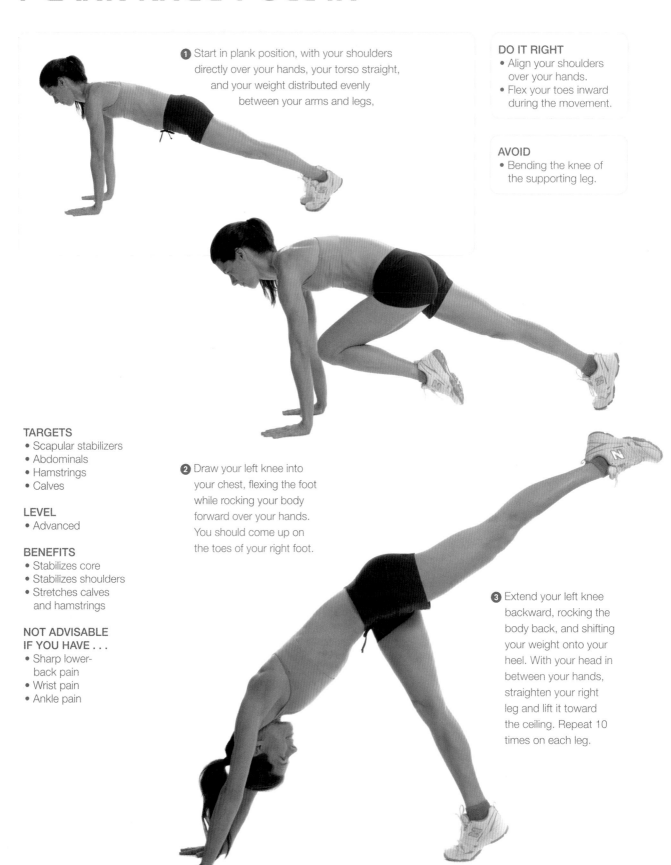

❶ Start in plank position, with your shoulders directly over your hands, your torso straight, and your weight distributed evenly between your arms and legs,

**DO IT RIGHT**
- Align your shoulders over your hands.
- Flex your toes inward during the movement.

**AVOID**
- Bending the knee of the supporting leg.

**TARGETS**
- Scapular stabilizers
- Abdominals
- Hamstrings
- Calves

**LEVEL**
- Advanced

**BENEFITS**
- Stabilizes core
- Stabilizes shoulders
- Stretches calves and hamstrings

**NOT ADVISABLE IF YOU HAVE . . .**
- Sharp lower-back pain
- Wrist pain
- Ankle pain

❷ Draw your left knee into your chest, flexing the foot while rocking your body forward over your hands. You should come up on the toes of your right foot.

❸ Extend your left knee backward, rocking the body back, and shifting your weight onto your heel. With your head in between your hands, straighten your right leg and lift it toward the ceiling. Repeat 10 times on each leg.

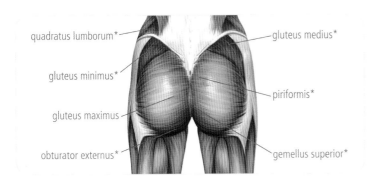

quadratus lumborum*
gluteus medius*
gluteus minimus*
piriformis*
gluteus maximus
obturator externus*
gemellus superior*

**ANNOTATION KEY**
**Black text indicates target muscles**
Gray text indicates other working muscles
* indicates deep muscles

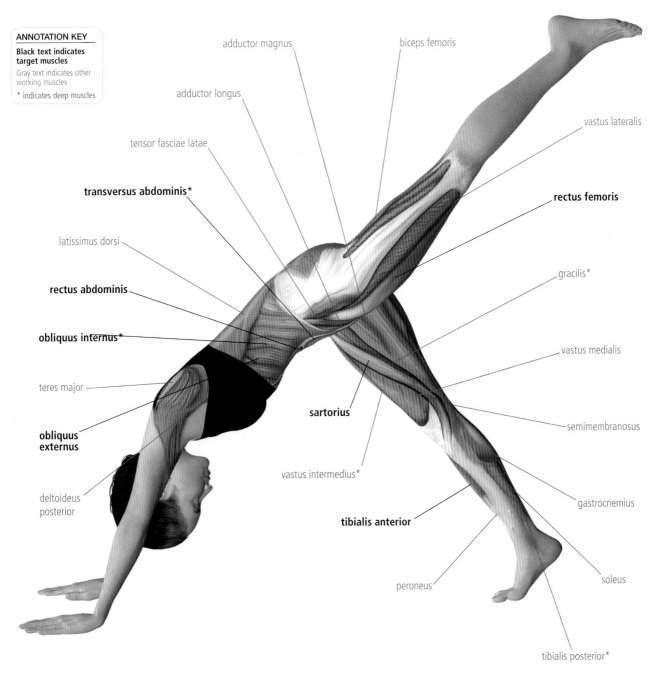

adductor magnus
biceps femoris
adductor longus
vastus lateralis
tensor fasciae latae
**transversus abdominis***
**rectus femoris**
latissimus dorsi
gracilis*
**rectus abdominis**
**obliquus internus***
vastus medialis
teres major
**obliquus externus**
sartorius
semimembranosus
vastus intermedius*
deltoideus posterior
gastrocnemius
**tibialis anterior**
peroneus
soleus
tibialis posterior*

# STANDING KNEE CRUNCH

**1** Stand tall with your left leg in front of the right, and extend your hands up toward the ceiling, your arms straight.

**AVOID**
• Tilting forward as you switch legs.

**DO IT RIGHT**
• Keep your standing leg straight as you raise up on your toes.
• Relax your shoulders as you pull your arms down for the crunch.
• Flex the toes of your raised leg.

**TARGETS**
• Pelvic and core stabilizers
• Abdominals
• Gluteal area

**LEVEL**
• Intermediate

**BENEFITS**
• Strengthens core
• Strengthens calves and gluteal muscles
• Improves balance

**NOT ADVISABLE IF YOU HAVE . . .**
• Knee pain

**2** Shift your weight onto your left foot, and raise your right knee to the height of your hips. Simultaneously go up on the toes of your left leg, while pulling your elbows down by your sides, your hands making fists. This creates the crunch.

**3** Pause at the top of the movement, and then return to the starting position. Repeat the sequence with your right leg as the standing leg. Repeat 10 times on each leg.

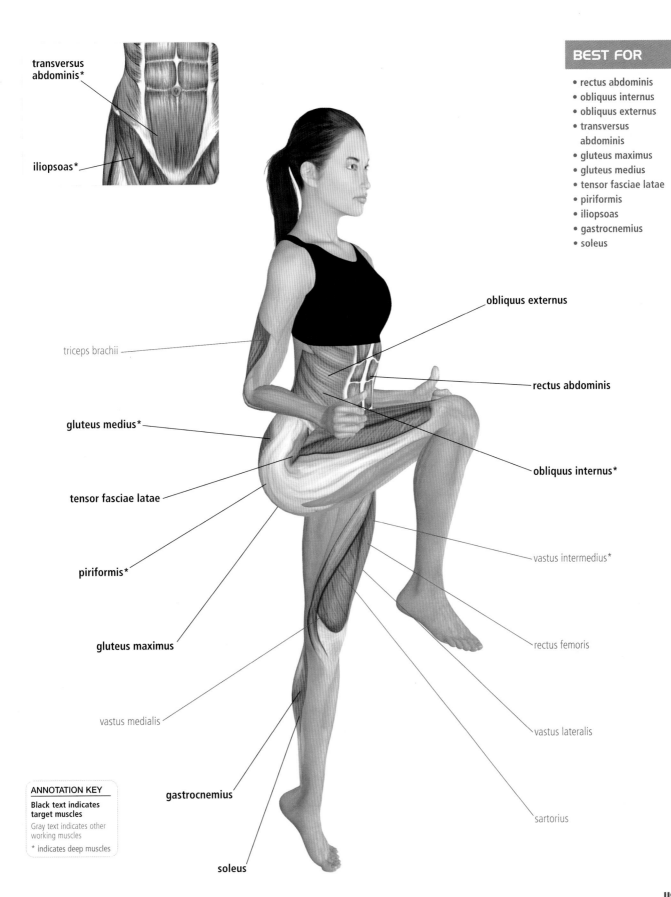

transversus abdominis*

iliopsoas*

**BEST FOR**

- rectus abdominis
- obliquus internus
- obliquus externus
- transversus abdominis
- gluteus maximus
- gluteus medius
- tensor fasciae latae
- piriformis
- iliopsoas
- gastrocnemius
- soleus

obliquus externus

triceps brachii

rectus abdominis

gluteus medius*

obliquus internus*

tensor fasciae latae

vastus intermedius*

piriformis*

gluteus maximus

rectus femoris

vastus medialis

vastus lateralis

gastrocnemius

sartorius

**ANNOTATION KEY**

**Black text indicates target muscles**

Gray text indicates other working muscles

* indicates deep muscles

soleus

# ILIOTIBIAL BAND RELEASE

**1** Lie on your left side, with the foam roller placed under the middle of your thigh. Support your torso with your left forearm on the floor.

**2** Bend your left leg and cross it in front of your right, so that your knee is pointed upward. Place your left foot flat on the floor.

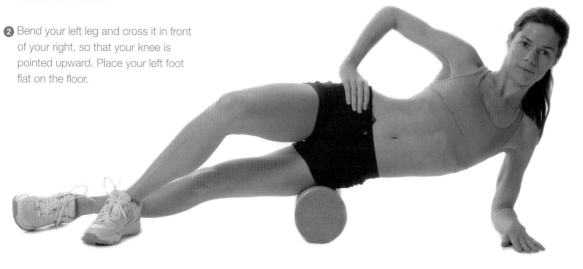

### TARGETS
- Iliotibial band
- Lateral thigh muscles
- Scapular stabilizers

### LEVEL
- Intermediate

### BENEFITS
- Releases the iliotibial band—this may be uncomfortable at first, but will become easier with repetition
- Strengthens the scapular stabilizers and lateral trunk muscles

### NOT ADVISABLE IF YOU HAVE . . .
- Shoulder pain
- Back pain

**3** Pulling with your shoulder and pushing with your supporting leg, roll back and forth along the side of your thigh. Adjust the placement of your arm as you make your motion bigger.

**4** Repeat 15 times on each side.

### DO IT RIGHT
- Relax your shoulders throughout the exercise.
- Press your hands and forearms firmly into the floor.

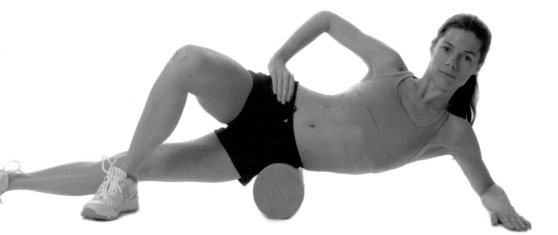

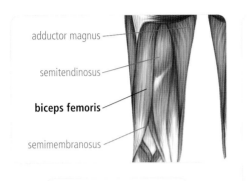

adductor magnus

semitendinosus

**biceps femoris**

semimembranosus

### AVOID
• Allowing your shoulders
  to lift toward your ears.

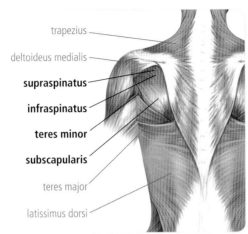

trapezius

deltoideus medialis

**supraspinatus**

**infraspinatus**

**teres minor**

**subscapularis**

teres major

latissimus dorsi

## BEST FOR
• tractus iliotibialis
• rectus femoris
• vastus medialis
• vastus intermedius
• vastus lateralis
• biceps femoris
• infraspinatus
• supraspinatus
• teres minor
• subscapularis

**ANNOTATION KEY**
**Black text indicates target muscles**
Gray text indicates other working muscles
\* indicates deep muscles

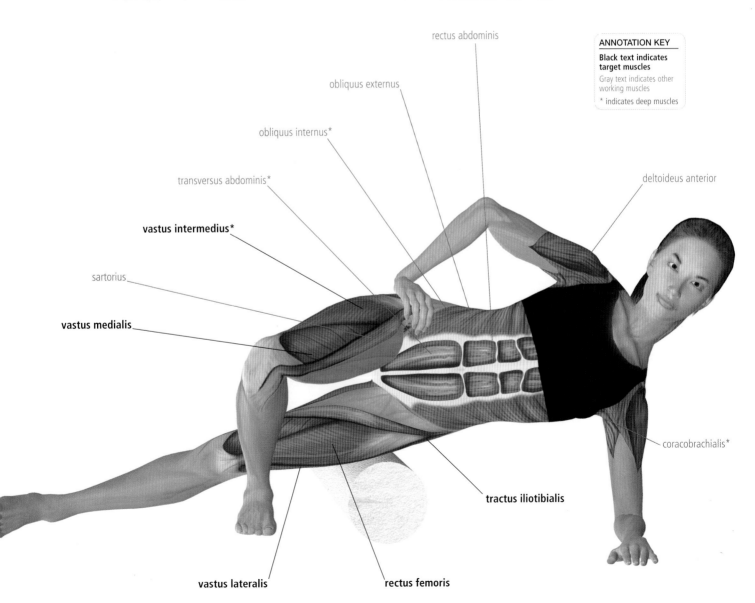

rectus abdominis

obliquus externus

obliquus internus*

transversus abdominis*

vastus intermedius*

sartorius

**vastus medialis**

deltoideus anterior

coracobrachialis*

**tractus iliotibialis**

**vastus lateralis**     **rectus femoris**

# BRIDGE WITH LEG LIFT

**1** Lie on your back, with the roller under your shoulders. Your buttocks should be on the floor, with your knees bent, and feet flat on the floor.

**DO IT RIGHT**
- Keep your extended leg straight.

**TARGETS**
- Gluteal area
- Hamstrings

**LEVEL**
- Advanced

**BENEFITS**
- Improves pelvic stabilization
- Strengthens gluteal muscles
- Strengthens hamstrings

**NOT ADVISABLE IF YOU HAVE . . .**
- Hamstring injury
- Lower-back pain
- Ankle pain

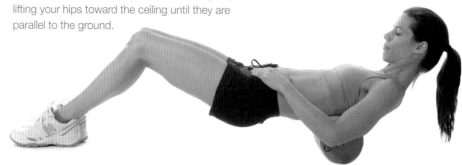

**2** Press into the floor with your feet and bridge up, lifting your hips toward the ceiling until they are parallel to the ground.

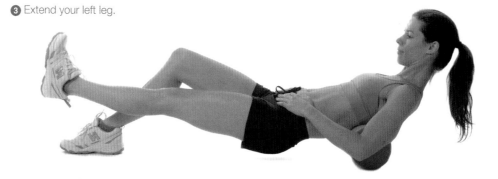

**3** Extend your left leg.

**4** Raise your left leg up to the height of your knees. Keeping your leg straight and the roller still, raise and lower your hips.

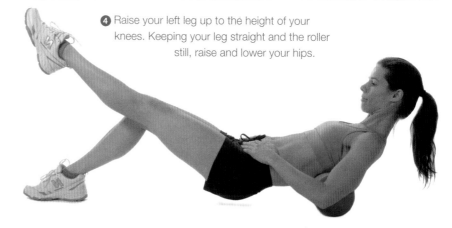

# BRIDGE WITH LEG LIFT • TARGET: SECONDARY MUSCLES

**5** Return to step 2 and repeat step 3 and step 4 with the right leg.

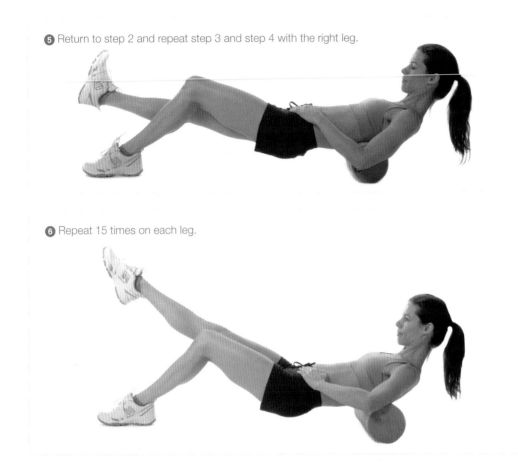

**6** Repeat 15 times on each leg.

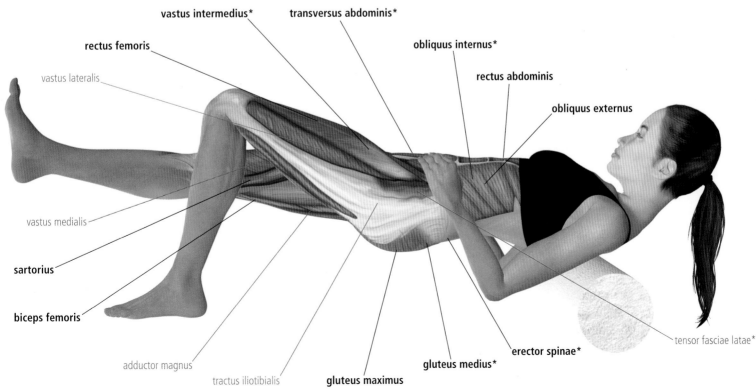

vastus intermedius*

transversus abdominis*

rectus femoris

obliquus internus*

rectus abdominis

vastus lateralis

obliquus externus

vastus medialis

sartorius

biceps femoris

tensor fasciae latae*

adductor magnus

erector spinae*

tractus iliotibialis

gluteus medius*

gluteus maximus

# PUSH-UP

❶ From a standing position, walk your hands out until they are directly beneath your shoulders in a high plank position.

❷ Inhale, and set your body by drawing your abdominals to your spine. Squeeze your buttocks and legs together and stretch out of your heels, bringing your body into a straight line.

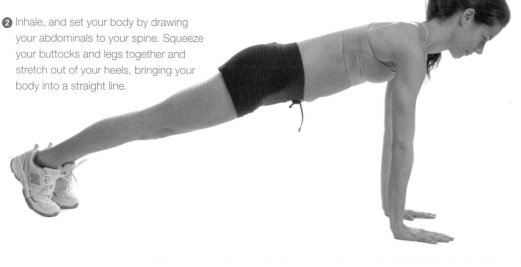

❸ Exhale and inhale as you bend your elbows and lower your body toward the floor.

**TARGETS**
• Chest
• Upper arms

**LEVEL**
• Beginner

**BENEFITS**
• Strengthens the core stabilizers, shoulders, back, buttocks, and pectoral muscles

**NOT ADVISABLE IF YOU HAVE . . .**
• Shoulder issues
• Wrist pain
• Lower-back pain

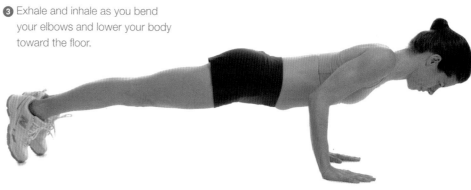

❹ Push upward to return to plank position. Keep your elbows close to your body. Repeat eight times.

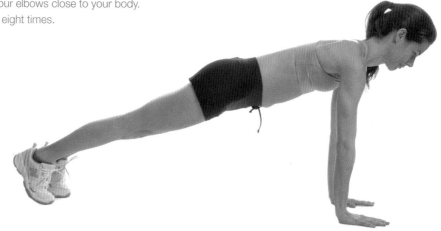

## DO IT RIGHT
- Relax your neck, keeping it long as you perform the upward movement.
- Squeeze your glutes as you scoop in your abdominals for stability.

## AVOID
- Allowing your shoulders to lift toward your ears.

### ANNOTATION KEY
**Black text indicates target muscles**
Gray text indicates other working muscles
* indicates deep muscles

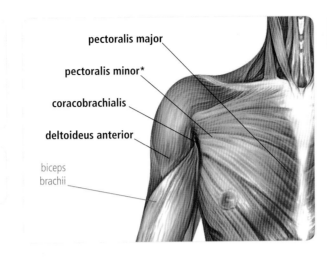

pectoralis major
pectoralis minor*
coracobrachialis
deltoideus anterior
biceps brachii

### BEST FOR
- triceps brachii
- pectoralis major
- pectoralis minor
- coracobrachialis
- deltoideus anterior
- rectus abdominis
- transversus abdominis
- obliquus externus
- obliquus internus
- trapezius

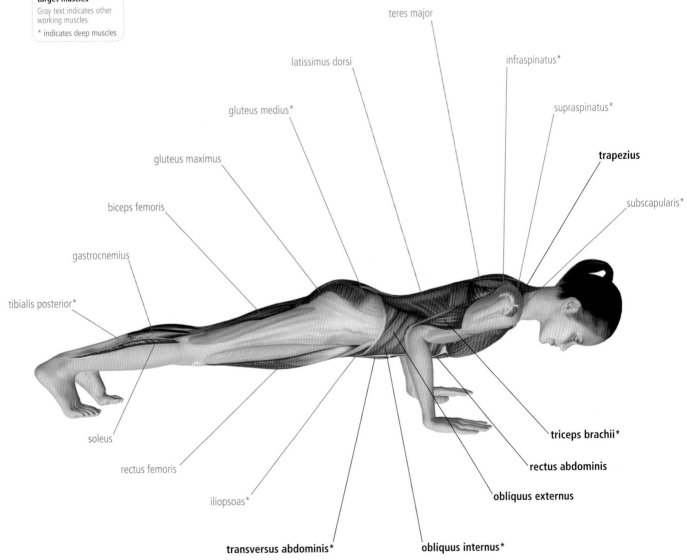

teres major
latissimus dorsi
gluteus medius*
gluteus maximus
biceps femoris
gastrocnemius
tibialis posterior*
soleus
rectus femoris
iliopsoas*
transversus abdominis*
obliquus internus*
infraspinatus*
supraspinatus*
**trapezius**
subscapularis*
**triceps brachii***
**rectus abdominis**
**obliquus externus**

# SWISS BALL PUSH-UP

① Place your toes on top of an exercise ball, and walk your arms out until your legs are fully extended and your body forms a straight line from shoulders to feet, your hands shoulder-width apart.

### DO IT RIGHT
• Form a straight plane from neck to ankles.
• Inhale as you lower your torso, and exhale as you press back up.

### AVOID
• Arching your back during the exercise.
• Rotating your hips.
• Locking your elbows.
• Allowing your lower back and hips to droop—this can place increased pressure on the lumbar vertebrae and could lead to a back injury.

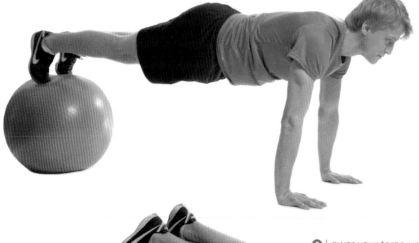

② Lower your torso until your chest almost touches the floor.

### TARGETS
• Chest
• Shoulders
• Upper Arms

### LEVEL
• Intermediate

### BENEFITS
• Strengthens shoulders
• Stabilizes core
• Strengthens abdominals

### NOT ADVISABLE IF YOU HAVE . . .
• Wrist pain
• Lower-back pain
• Shoulder instability

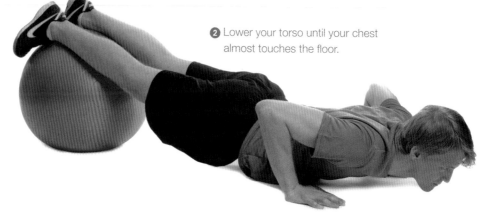

③ Press your upper body back up to the starting position and squeeze your chest. Pause at the contracted position, and repeat the flexing and extending at your elbows for three sets of 10 repetitions.

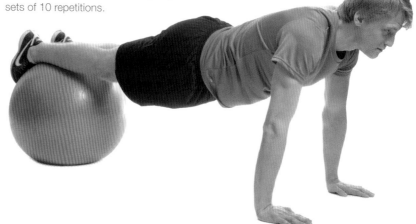

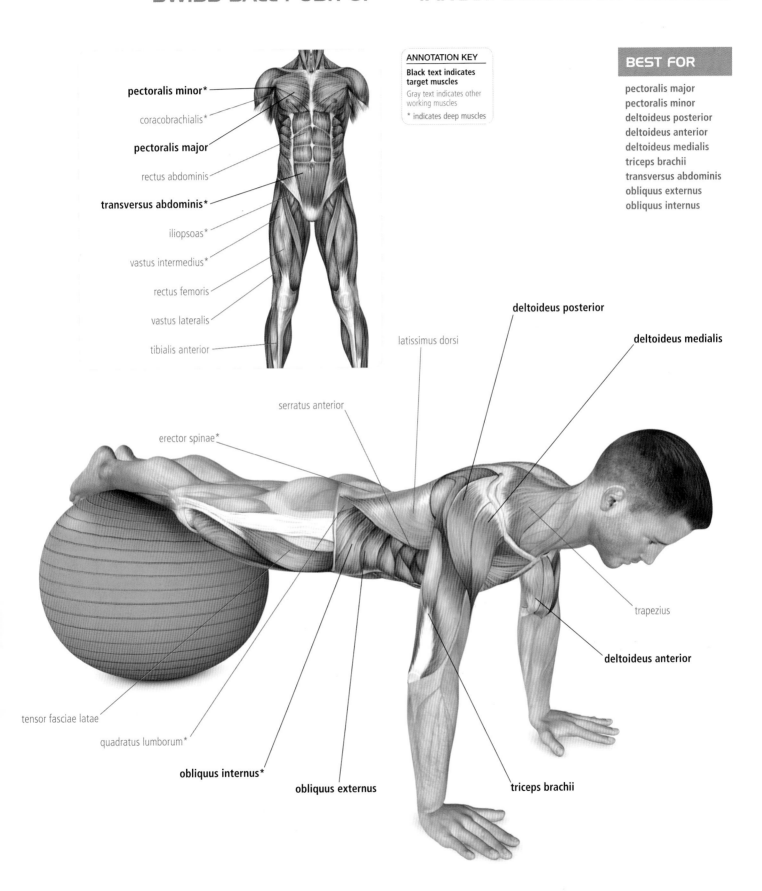

**ANNOTATION KEY**

**Black text indicates target muscles**
Gray text indicates other working muscles
* indicates deep muscles

**BEST FOR**

pectoralis major
pectoralis minor
deltoideus posterior
deltoideus anterior
deltoideus medialis
triceps brachii
transversus abdominis
obliquus externus
obliquus internus

**pectoralis minor***

coracobrachialis*

**pectoralis major**

rectus abdominis

**transversus abdominis***

iliopsoas*

vastus intermedius*

rectus femoris

vastus lateralis

tibialis anterior

latissimus dorsi

**deltoideus posterior**

**deltoideus medialis**

serratus anterior

erector spinae*

trapezius

**deltoideus anterior**

tensor fasciae latae

quadratus lumborum*

**obliquus internus***

**obliquus externus**

**triceps brachii**

# SWISS BALL WALKOUT

1 Lie prone on a Swiss ball, with your hips over the center of the ball as you support your weight on your arms. Your hands should be directly below your shoulders.

**DO IT RIGHT**
• Form a straight plane from neck to ankles.
• Activate your abdominals as you straighten your back.

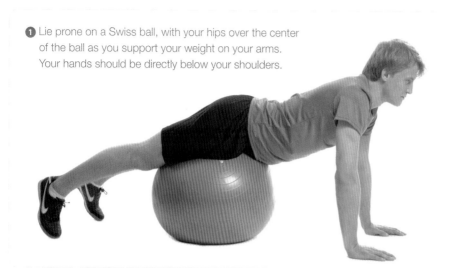

2 Lift, reach, and place your left hand forward, rolling the ball underneath you until it reaches your feet.

**TARGETS**
• Shoulders
• Upper back
• Abdominals

**LEVEL**
• Intermediate

**BENEFITS**
• Strengthens shoulders
• Stabilizes core
• Strengthens abdominals

**NOT ADVISABLE IF YOU HAVE . . .**
• Wrist pain
• Lower-back pain
• Shoulder instability

3 Hold for 5 seconds, and then walk your hands backward, rolling the ball back underneath you until you reach the starting position.

4 Repeat the entire sequence five times.

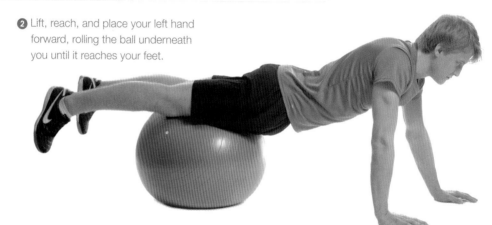

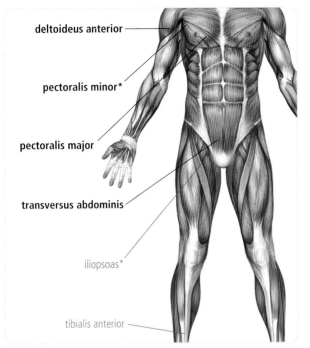

deltoideus anterior

pectoralis minor*

pectoralis major

transversus abdominis

iliopsoas*

tibialis anterior

## AVOID
- Arching your back during the exercise.
- Allowing your hips to rotate.
- Locking your elbows.
- Reaching too far forward — start with a short position reach and progressively increase the length as you gain stability.

## BEST FOR
- deltoideus anterior
- deltoideus medialis
- deltoideus posterior
- transversus abdominis
- triceps brachii
- pectoralis major
- pectoralis minor

### ANNOTATION KEY
**Black text indicates target muscles**
Gray text indicates other working muscles
* indicates deep muscles

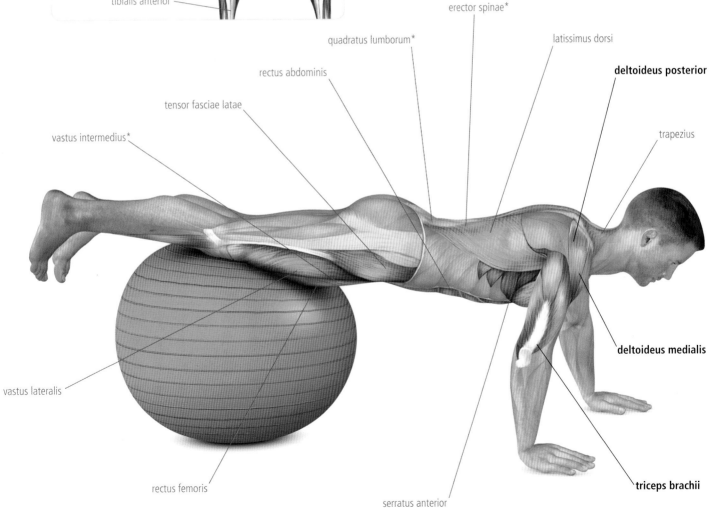

vastus intermedius*

tensor fasciae latae

rectus abdominis

quadratus lumborum*

erector spinae*

latissimus dorsi

**deltoideus posterior**

trapezius

**deltoideus medialis**

vastus lateralis

rectus femoris

serratus anterior

**triceps brachii**

# SWISS BALL EXTENSION

① Lie prone over a Swiss ball, with your upper chest and head hanging off the edge of the ball.

**DO IT RIGHT**
- Engage your glutes and thighs throughout the exercise.
- Keep the muscles of your lower body taut.
- Keep your head in neutral position.
- Maintain a wide base for extra balance.

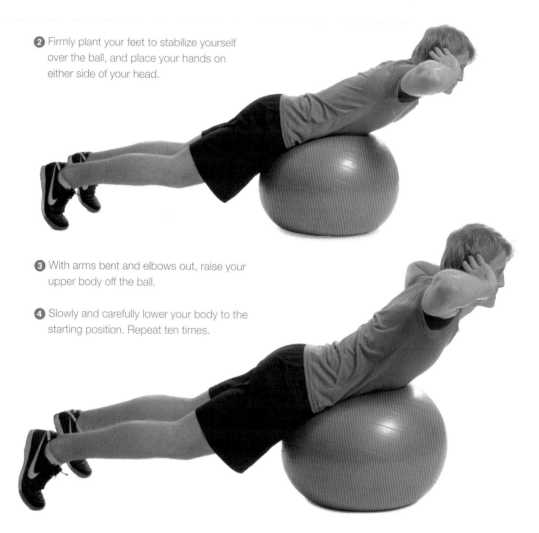

② Firmly plant your feet to stabilize yourself over the ball, and place your hands on either side of your head.

**TARGETS**
- Middle back
- Lower back

**LEVEL**
- Advanced

**BENEFITS**
- Stabilizes core
- Strengthens back extensor muscles
- Strengthens abdominals

**NOT ADVISABLE IF YOU HAVE . . .**
- Neck issues
- Lower-back pain

③ With arms bent and elbows out, raise your upper body off the ball.

④ Slowly and carefully lower your body to the starting position. Repeat ten times.

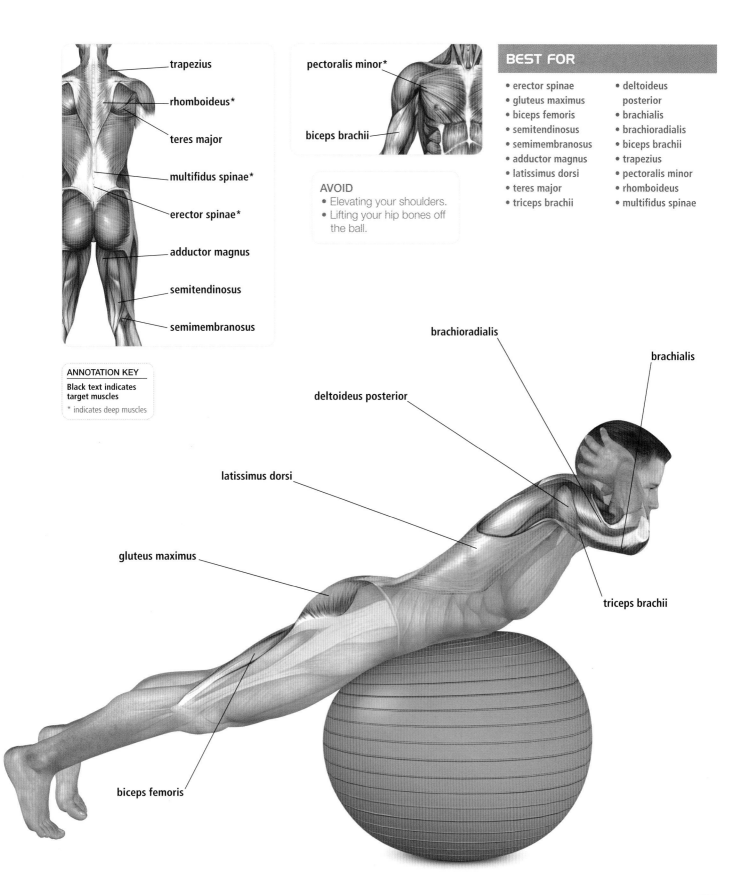

trapezius

rhomboideus*

teres major

multifidus spinae*

erector spinae*

adductor magnus

semitendinosus

semimembranosus

pectoralis minor*

biceps brachii

## BEST FOR

- erector spinae
- gluteus maximus
- biceps femoris
- semitendinosus
- semimembranosus
- adductor magnus
- latissimus dorsi
- teres major
- triceps brachii

- deltoideus posterior
- brachialis
- brachioradialis
- biceps brachii
- trapezius
- pectoralis minor
- rhomboideus
- multifidus spinae

## AVOID
- Elevating your shoulders.
- Lifting your hip bones off the ball.

## ANNOTATION KEY

Black text indicates target muscles

* indicates deep muscles

brachioradialis

brachialis

deltoideus posterior

latissimus dorsi

gluteus maximus

triceps brachii

biceps femoris

# BACKWARD BALL STRETCH

### DO IT RIGHT
- Maintain good balance throughout the stretch.
- Move slowly and in a controlled manner.
- Keep your head on the ball until you have dropped your knees all the way down as you release from the stretch.

### AVOID
- Allowing the ball to shift to the side.
- Holding the extended position for too long, or until you feel dizzy.

### TARGETS
- Thoracic and upper-lumbar spine
- Abdominals

### LEVEL
- Advanced

### BENEFITS
- Stretches thoracic spine
- Increases spinal extension
- Stretches abdominals and large back muscles

### NOT ADVISABLE IF YOU HAVE . . .
- Lower-back pain
- Balancing difficulty

**①** Sit on a Swiss ball in a well-balanced, neutral position, with your hips directly over the center of the ball.

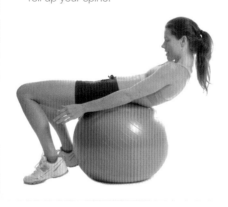

**②** While maintaining good balance, begin to extend your arms behind you.

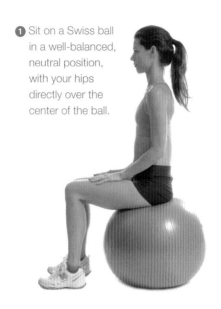

**③** Walk your feet forward, allowing the ball to roll up your spine.

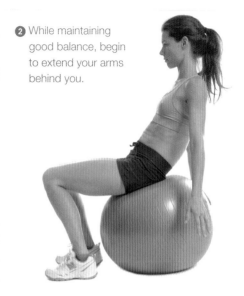

**④** As your hands touch the floor, extend your legs as far forward as you comfortably can. Hold this position for 10 seconds.

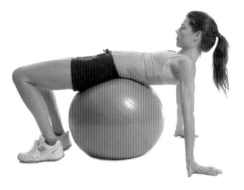

**⑤** To deepen the stretch, extend your arms, and walk your legs and hands closer to the ball. Hold this position for 10 seconds.

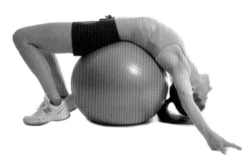

**⑥** To release the stretch, bend your knees, drop your hips to the floor, lift your head off the ball, and then walk back to the starting position.

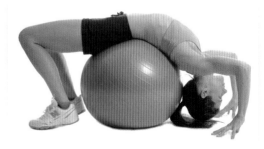

## MODIFICATION

**Harder:** Follow step 1, and then rather then reaching behind you, extend your arms upward as your walk your feet forward and roll backward on the ball.

latissimus dorsi

quadratus lumborum*

***ligamentum longitudinale anterius***

gluteus medius*

quadratus femoris*

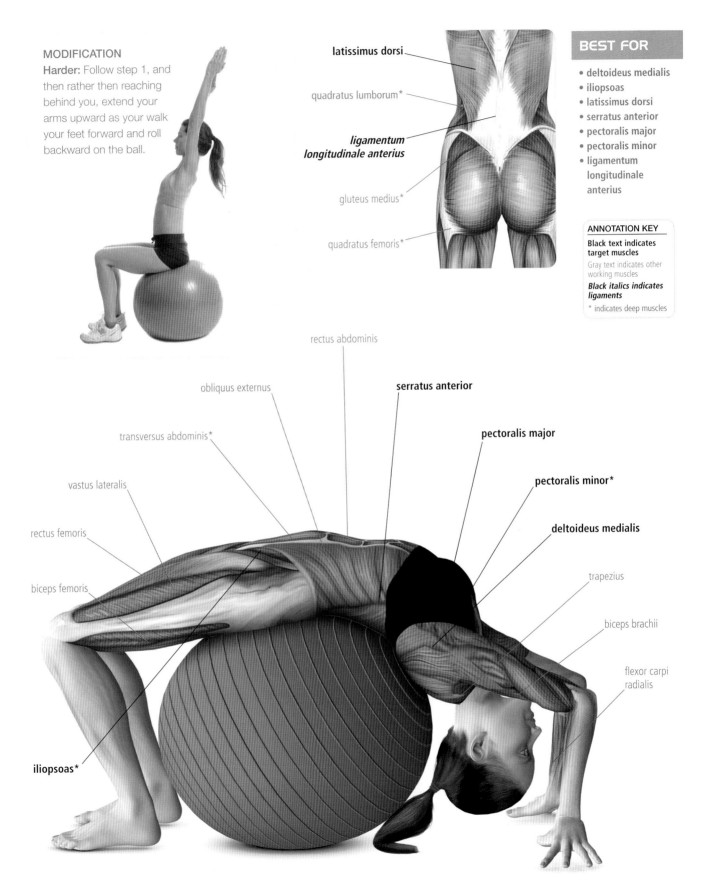

rectus abdominis

obliquus externus

**serratus anterior**

transversus abdominis*

**pectoralis major**

vastus lateralis

**pectoralis minor***

rectus femoris

**deltoideus medialis**

biceps femoris

trapezius

biceps brachii

flexor carpi radialis

**iliopsoas***

# BICEPS CURL

❶ Stand upright with the resistance band beneath your feet. Your arms should be very slightly bent as you hold both handles of the resistance band in your hands, palms forward.

**DO IT RIGHT**
• Keep your elbows at your sides.

❷ Curl the resistance band upward toward your shoulders.

❸ Lower and repeat, completing three sets of 15.

**TARGETS**
• Upper arms

**LEVEL**
• Beginner

**BENEFITS**
• Strengthens and tones biceps

**NOT ADVISABLE IF YOU HAVE . . .**
• Wrist or elbow pain

**AVOID**
• Rushing through the exercise.

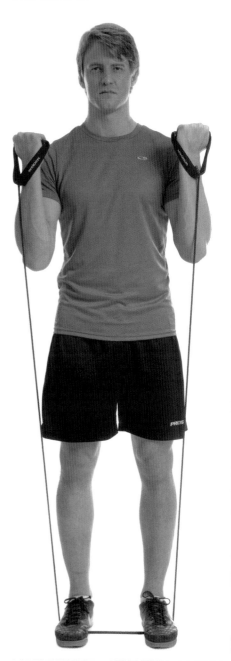

**BEST FOR**

• biceps brachii

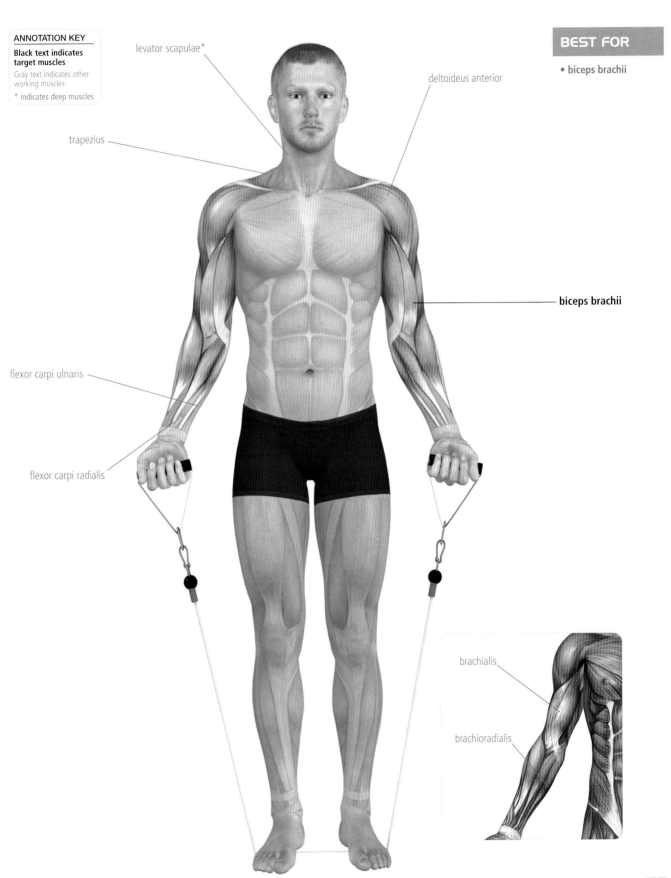

levator scapulae*

deltoideus anterior

trapezius

biceps brachii

flexor carpi ulnaris

flexor carpi radialis

brachialis

brachioradialis

# SWISS BALL SHOULDER PRESS

**1** Sit on a Swiss ball in a well-balanced, neutral position, with your hips directly over the center of the ball, grasping a dumbbell in each hand. Hold one to each side of your shoulders with your elbows below wrists.

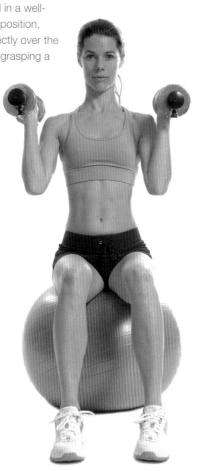

**BEST FOR**

• deltoideus anterior

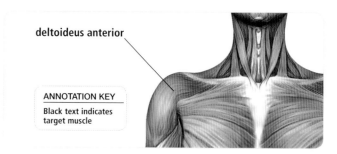

deltoideus anterior

**ANNOTATION KEY**
Black text indicates target muscle

**2** Press the dumbbells upward until your arms are fully extended overhead.

**3** Lower to sides of shoulders and repeat 10 to 15 repetitions.

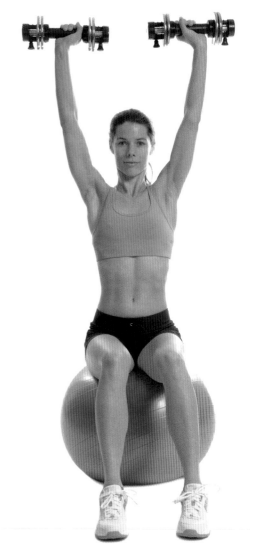

**TARGETS**
• Shoulders

**LEVEL**
• Beginner

**BENEFITS**
• Strengthens and tones front of shoulders

**NOT ADVISABLE IF YOU HAVE . . .**
• Shoulder issues
• Rotator cuff injury

**DO IT RIGHT**
• Pause at the top of the movement, and then lower to just above the start position, keeping tension on the muscles until the set is complete.
• Keep your elbows rigid without locking them at the top of the movement.

**AVOID**
• Tensing your neck.
• Wiggling or squirming in an effort to press the weights upward.

# TRICEPS EXTENSION

1. Stand with your legs and feet parallel and shoulder-width apart, grasping a dumbbell or hand weight in your right hand. Position the dumbbell over your head with your arm straight up or slightly back.

2. Lower the dumbbell behind your neck or shoulder while maintaining your upper arm's vertical position.

3. Extend your arm until straight. Repeat for 10 to 15 repetitions.

4. Return to starting position, and repeat on the opposite side.

**DO IT RIGHT**
- Let the weight pull your arm back slightly to maintain full shoulder flexion.
- Keep your forearm in line with your ear throughout the exercise.
- Place your nonmoving hand just under your ribs to stabilize your shoulder.

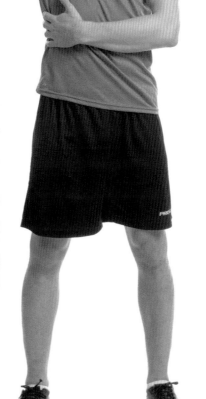

triceps brachii

**ANNOTATION KEY**
Black text indicates target muscle

**AVOID**
- Dropping your elbow back or forward.

**BEST FOR**

- triceps brachii

**TARGETS**
- Upper arms

**LEVEL**
- Beginner

**BENEFITS**
- Strengthens and tones upper arms

**NOT ADVISABLE IF YOU HAVE . . .**
- Shoulder issues
- Rotator cuff injury

# LATERAL SHOULDER RAISE

**1** Holding a dumbbell in each hand, stand with your feet parallel and shoulder width apart, your knees slightly bent. Bend your elbow slightly and face your palms in toward the body.

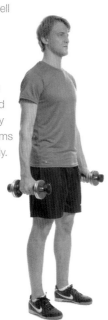

**2** Extend both arms out to the sides to shoulder height.

**3** Slowly lower the dumbbells back to the starting position. Repeat, completing three sets of 10.

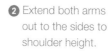

**AVOID**
- Using momentum to lift the dumbbells.
- Dropping your elbows lower than your wrists— this will make the front deltoids the primary movers instead of the lateral deltoids.

**TARGETS**
- Shoulders

**LEVEL**
- Beginner

**BENEFITS**
- Strengthens medial deltoids
- Strengthens thoracic spine

**NOT ADVISABLE IF YOU HAVE . . .**
- Acute rotator cuff injury

**MODIFICATION**
**Similar level of difficulty:** Secure a resistance band under both feet. Stand with feet shoulder-width apart, and then with a an end in each hand, extend both arms out to the sides to shoulder height. Slowly lower back to the starting position.

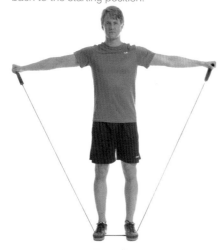

**DO IT RIGHT**
- Keep your elbows in a fixed and slightly bent position throughout the movement.
- Position your elbows directly lateral to your shoulders at the top of the movement.
- Exhale as you lift the dumbbells, and inhale as you lower them.
- Keep your chest elevated.
- Keep your shoulders down.

# LATERAL SHOULDER RAISE • TARGET: SECONDARY MUSCLES

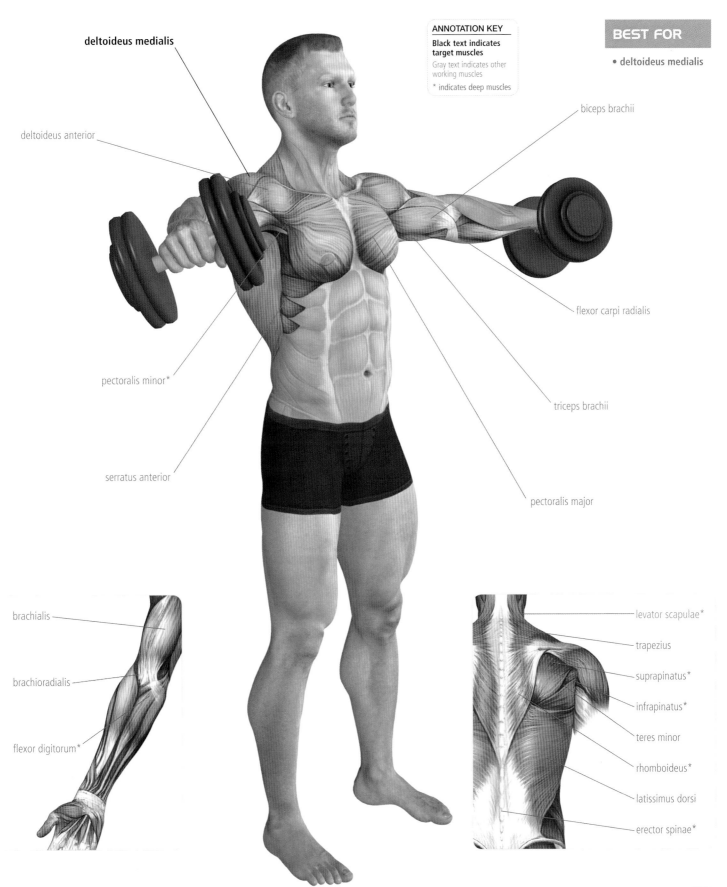

deltoideus medialis

deltoideus anterior

pectoralis minor*

serratus anterior

**BEST FOR**

• deltoideus medialis

biceps brachii

flexor carpi radialis

triceps brachii

pectoralis major

brachialis

brachioradialis

flexor digitorum*

levator scapulae*

trapezius

suprapinatus*

infrapinatus*

teres minor

rhomboideus*

latissimus dorsi

erector spinae*

# SHOULDER RAISE AND PULL

**1** Holding a dumbbell or hand weight in each hand, stand with your legs and feet parallel and shoulder-width apart. Bend your knees very slightly and tuck your pelvis slightly forward, lift your chest, and press your shoulders downward and back.

**DO IT RIGHT**
• Keep a slight bend in your elbow as you lift upward to avoid stress on the joints.

**2** Bring your arms up to a 90-degree angle from the front of the body.

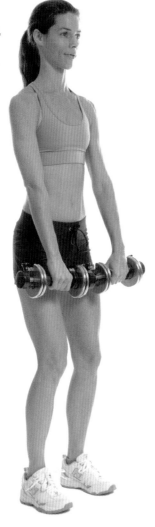

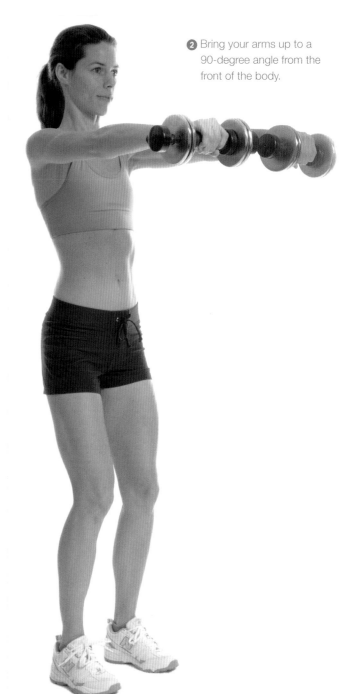

**TARGETS**
• Shoulders

**LEVEL**
• Beginner

**BENEFITS**
• Strengthens shoulders

**NOT ADVISABLE IF YOU HAVE . . .**
• Shoulder issues
• Rotator cuff injury

**AVOID**
• Raising your elbows or the weight higher than your shoulders.

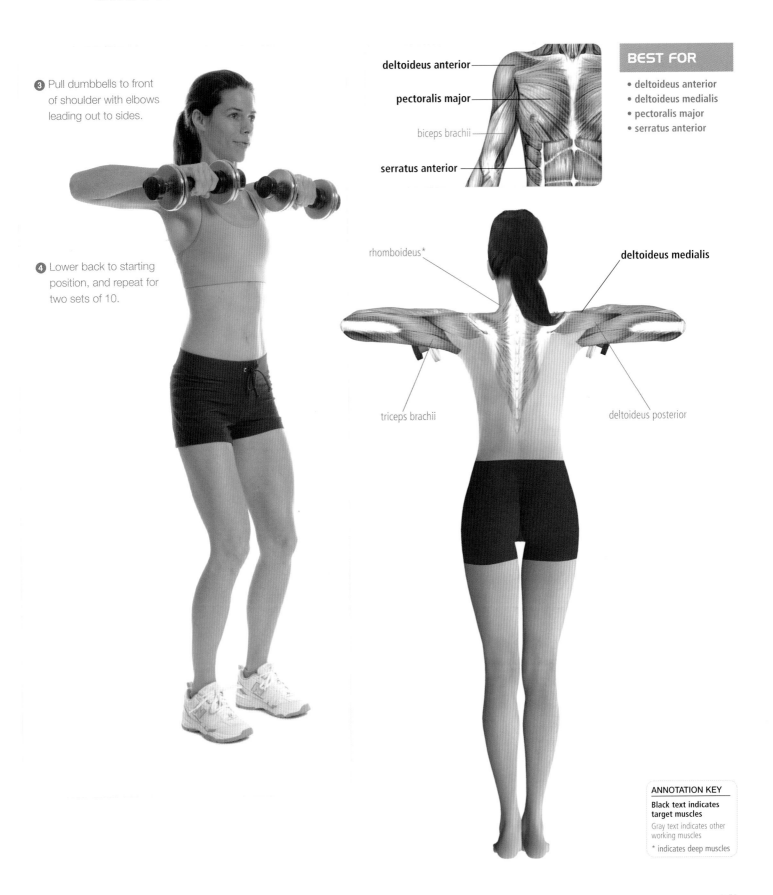

**③** Pull dumbbells to front of shoulder with elbows leading out to sides.

**④** Lower back to starting position, and repeat for two sets of 10.

deltoideus anterior

pectoralis major

biceps brachii

serratus anterior

**BEST FOR**

- deltoideus anterior
- deltoideus medialis
- pectoralis major
- serratus anterior

rhomboideus*

deltoideus medialis

triceps brachii

deltoideus posterior

**ANNOTATION KEY**

**Black text indicates target muscles**

Gray text indicates other working muscles

* indicates deep muscles

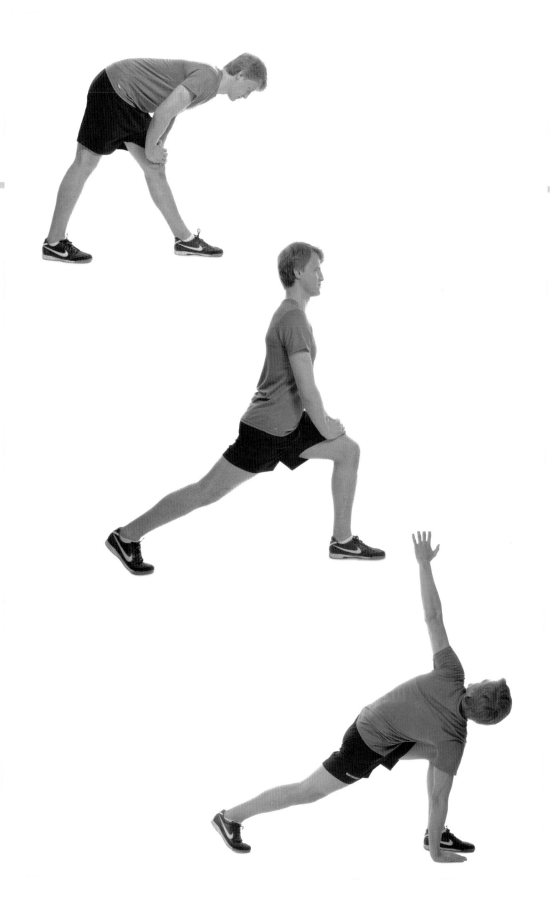

# PUT IT ALL TOGETHER:
# WORKOUTS

Once you have gone through the stretching and strengthening

exercises in this book and practiced executing them properly, your

next step is to put these moves together. The following sequences are

just samples of the many ways that you can combine these exercises

to create running warm-ups, cool-downs, and all-over strengthening

workouts, as well as ones that target the upper and lower body. They

provide flexible frameworks that you can adapt to accommodate

your specific fitness level or area of concern—if you want to avoid a

certain exercise in any one of them, simply substitute another that

has a similar benefit. Try the workouts featured here, and then flip

through the exercises and create your own stretching routines and

strengthening workouts to suit your individual goals.

# BEGINNER STRETCHING ROUTINE

Perform this series of stretches before you run and as a cool-down post-run.

**1 Forward Lunge**

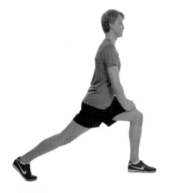

pages 28–29

**2 Straight-Leg Lunge**

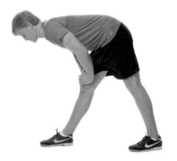

pages 32–33

**3 Wide-Legged Forward Bend**

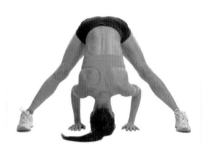

pages 34–35

**4 Knee-to-Chest Hug**

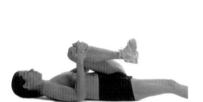

pages 40–41

**5 Unilateral Leg Raise**

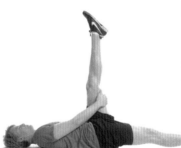

pages 42–43

**6 Cobra Stretch**

pages 48–49

**7 Hip/Iliotibial Band Stretch**

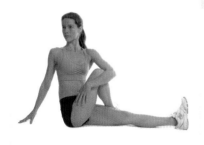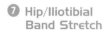

pages 52–53

**8 Gastrocnemius Stretch**

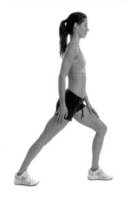

page 58

**9 Soleus Stretch**

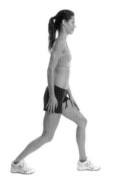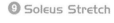

page 59

# INTERMEDIATE STRETCHING ROUTINE

Try these stretches before and after a run, adding new ones as you become more conditioned.

**①** Standing
Quadriceps Stretch

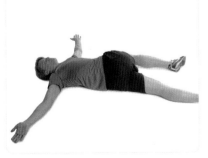

page 26

**②** Sprinter Stretch

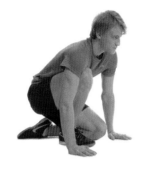

page 27

**③** Unilateral Seated
Forward Bend

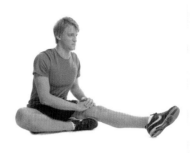

pages 36–37

**④** Supine Figure 4

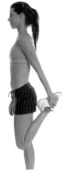

pages 44–45

**⑤** Side-Lying Knee Bend

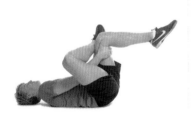

pages 46–47

**⑥** Side-Lying Rib Stretch

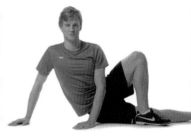

pages 50–51

**⑦** Pretzel Stretch

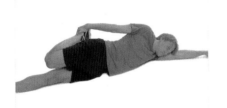

pages 54–55

**⑧** Heel-Drop/
Toe-Up Stretch

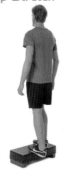

pages 56–57

**⑨** Iliotibial Band Stretch

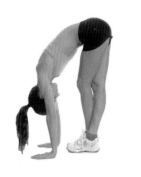

page 60

# ADVANCED STRETCHING ROUTINE

This balanced series of stretches works all of your primary running muscles.

**1** Bilateral Seated Forward Bend

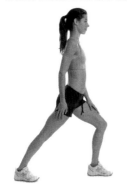

pages 38–39

**2** Standing Quadriceps Stretch

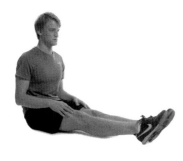

page 26

**3** Sprinter Stretch

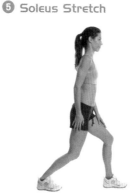

page 27

**4** Gastrocnemius Stretch

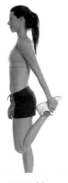

page 58

**5** Soleus Stretch

page 59

**6** Iliotibial Band Stretch

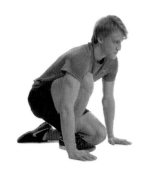

page 60

**7** Forward Lunge with Twist

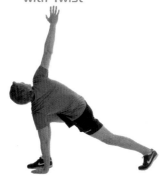

pages 30–31

**8** Resistance Band Tendon Stretch

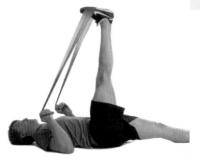

page 61

**9** Resistance Band Ankle Stretches

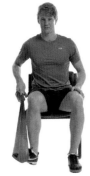

pages 62–63

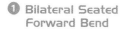
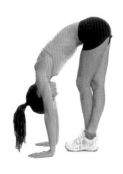

WORKOUTS

# BEGINNER STRENGTHENING WORKOUT

This series of exercises will help you begin building strength in the key running muscles.

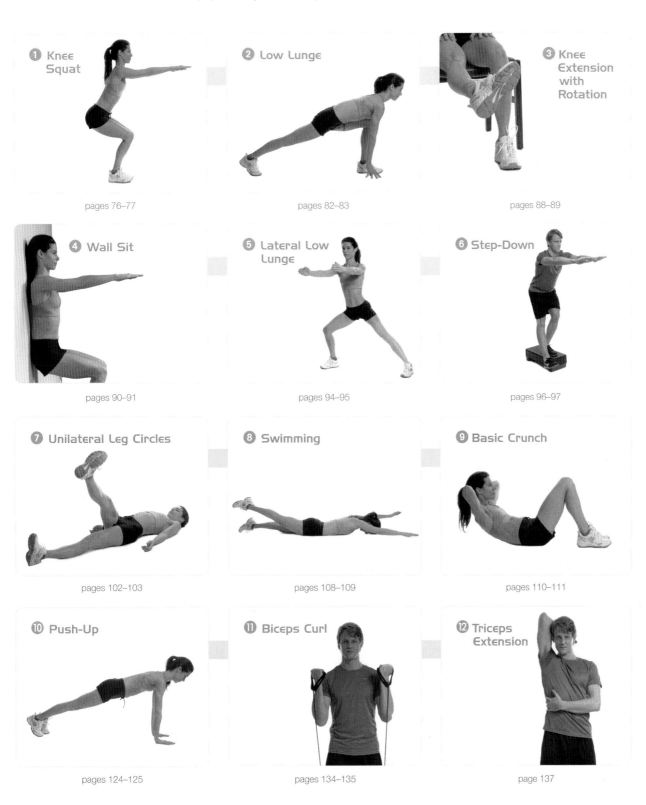

**1** Knee Squat

pages 76–77

**2** Low Lunge

pages 82–83

**3** Knee Extension with Rotation

pages 88–89

**4** Wall Sit

pages 90–91

**5** Lateral Low Lunge

pages 94–95

**6** Step-Down

pages 96–97

**7** Unilateral Leg Circles

pages 102–103

**8** Swimming

pages 108–109

**9** Basic Crunch

pages 110–111

**10** Push-Up

pages 124–125

**11** Biceps Curl

pages 134–135

**12** Triceps Extension

page 137

# INTERMEDIATE STRENGTHENING WORKOUT

When you start feeling the results of your workout and running regimen, try this series of exercises.

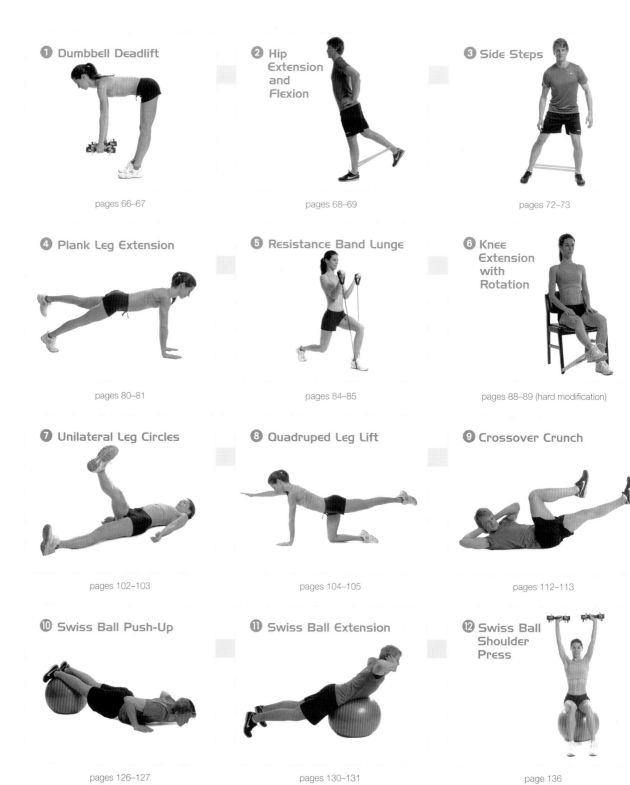

**1** Dumbbell Deadlift

pages 66–67

**2** Hip Extension and Flexion

pages 68–69

**3** Side Steps

pages 72–73

**4** Plank Leg Extension

pages 80–81

**5** Resistance Band Lunge

pages 84–85

**6** Knee Extension with Rotation

pages 88–89 (hard modification)

**7** Unilateral Leg Circles

pages 102–103

**8** Quadruped Leg Lift

pages 104–105

**9** Crossover Crunch

pages 112–113

**10** Swiss Ball Push-Up

pages 126–127

**11** Swiss Ball Extension

pages 130–131

**12** Swiss Ball Shoulder Press

page 136

# ADVANCED STRENGTHENING WORKOUT

Advanced runners can challenge themselves with this targeted set of muscle strengtheners.

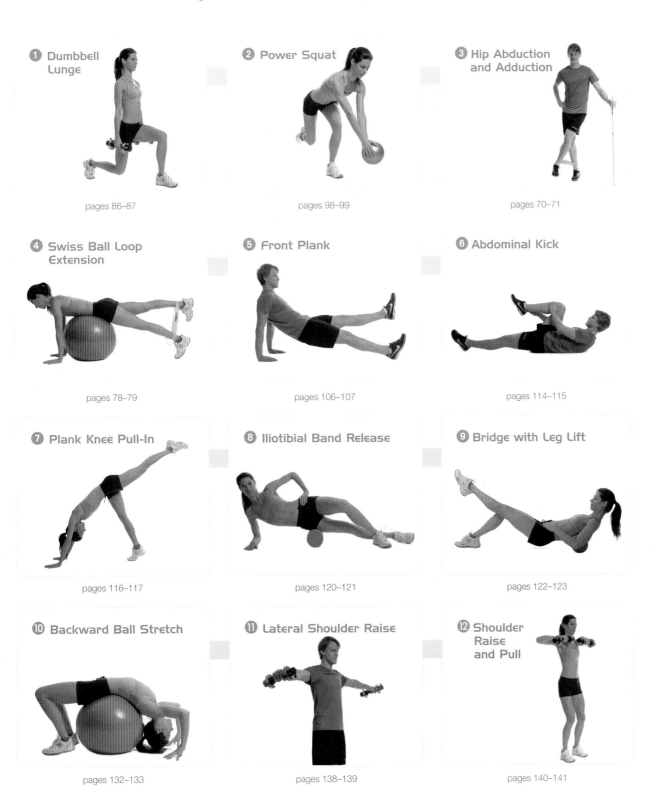

**1** Dumbbell Lunge

pages 86–87

**2** Power Squat

pages 98–99

**3** Hip Abduction and Adduction

pages 70–71

**4** Swiss Ball Loop Extension

pages 78–79

**5** Front Plank

pages 106–107

**6** Abdominal Kick

pages 114–115

**7** Plank Knee Pull-In

pages 116–117

**8** Iliotibial Band Release

pages 120–121

**9** Bridge with Leg Lift

pages 122–123

**10** Backward Ball Stretch

pages 132–133

**11** Lateral Shoulder Raise

pages 138–139

**12** Shoulder Raise and Pull

pages 140–141

# CORE FOCUS FOR RUNNERS

A strong core is essential for any athlete, so try this workout to enhance your running routine.

**1 Basic Crunch**

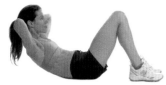

pages 110–111

**2 Standing Knee Crunch**

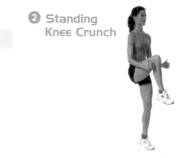

pages 118–119

**3 Swiss Ball Extension**

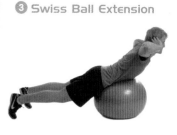

pages 130–131

**4 Swiss Ball Wall Sit**

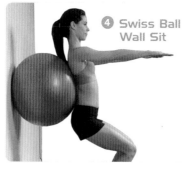

pages 92–93

**5 Swimming**

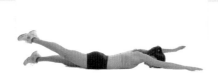

pages 108–109

**6 Abdominal Kick**

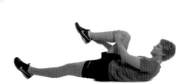

pages 114–115

**7 Quadruped Leg Lift**

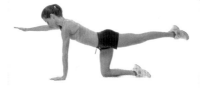

pages 104–105

**8 Iliotibial Band Release**

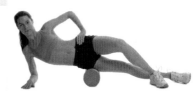

pages 120–121

**9 Crossover Crunch**

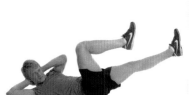

pages 112–113

**10 Plank Knee Pull-In**

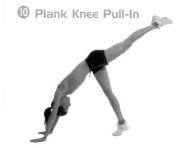

pages 116–117

**11 Bridge with Leg Lift**

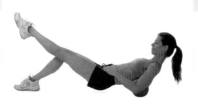

pages 122–123

**12 Front Plank**

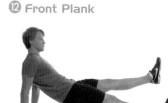

pages 106–107

# RUNNERS' FULL-BODY WORKOUT

This series offers a full-body workout that works both primary and secondary running muscles.

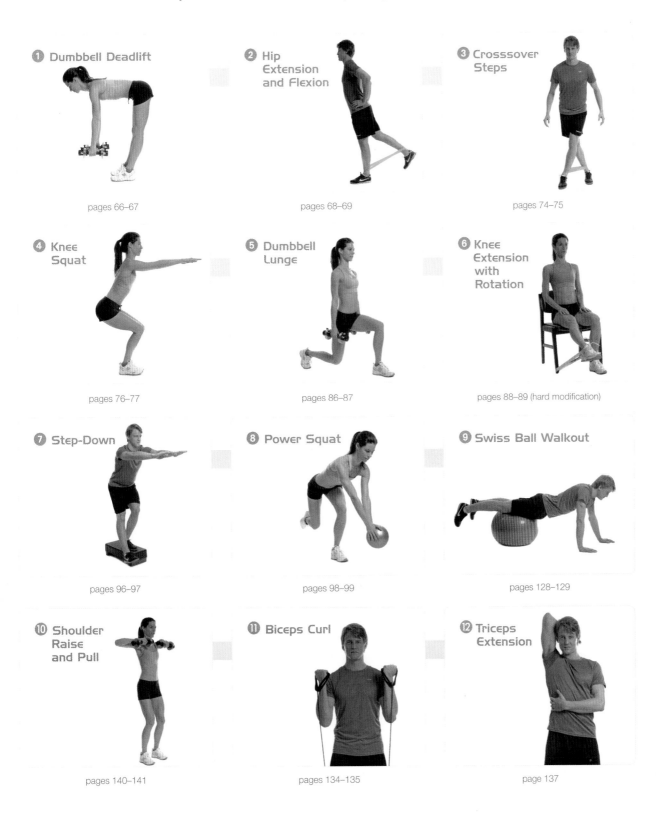

**1** Dumbbell Deadlift

pages 66–67

**2** Hip Extension and Flexion

pages 68–69

**3** Crosssover Steps

pages 74–75

**4** Knee Squat

pages 76–77

**5** Dumbbell Lunge

pages 86–87

**6** Knee Extension with Rotation

pages 88–89 (hard modification)

**7** Step-Down

pages 96–97

**8** Power Squat

pages 98–99

**9** Swiss Ball Walkout

pages 128–129

**10** Shoulder Raise and Pull

pages 140–141

**11** Biceps Curl

pages 134–135

**12** Triceps Extension

page 137

# GLOSSARY

## GENERAL TERMS

**abduction:** Movement away from the body.

**adduction:** Movement toward the body.

**aerobic step:** A portable step or platform with adjustable risers designed for cardiovascular exercising that also allows you to effectively work your calf muscles.

**agonist muscle:** See *antagonist muscle*.

**antagonist muscle:** A muscle working in opposition to another, called the *agonist*. Most muscles work in antagonistic pairs, with one muscle contracting as the other expands; for example, when the biceps brachii contracts, the triceps brachii relaxes.

**anterior:** Located in the front.

**cardiovascular exercise:** Any exercise that increases the heart rate, making oxygen and nutrient-rich blood available to working muscles.

**core:** Refers to the deep muscle layers that lie close to the spine and provide structural support for the entire body. The core is divisible into two groups: the major core and the minor core. The major muscles reside on the trunk and include the belly area and the mid and lower back. This area encompasses the pelvic floor muscles (levator ani, pubococcygeus, iliococcygeus, puborectalis, and coccygeus), the abdominals (rectus abdominis, transversus abdominis, obliquus externus, and obliquus internus), the spinal extensors (multifidus spinae, erector spinae, splenius, longissimus thoracis, and semispinalis), and the diaphragm. The minor core muscles include the latissimus dorsi, gluteus maximus, and trapezius. Minor core muscles assist the major muscles when the body engages in activities or movements that require added stability.

**crunch:** A common abdominal exercise that calls for curling the shoulders toward the pelvis while lying supine with hands behind the head and knees bent.

**curl:** An exercise movement, usually targeting the biceps brachii, that calls for a weight to be moved through an arc, in a "curling" motion.

**deadlift:** An exercise movement that calls for lifting a weight, such as a dumbbell, off the floor from a stabilized bent-over position.

**dumbbell:** A basic piece of equipment that consists of a short bar on which plates are secured. A person can use a dumbbell in one or both hands during an exercise. Most gyms offer dumbbells with the weight plates welded on and poundage indicated on the plates, but many dumbbells intended for home use come with removable plates that allow you to adjust the weight.

**extension:** The act of straightening.

**extensor muscle:** A muscle serving to extend a body part away from the body.

**flexion:** The bending of a joint.

**flexor muscle:** A muscle that decreases the angle between two bones, as when bending the arm at the elbow or raising the thigh toward the stomach.

**foam roller:** A tube that comes in a variety of sizes, materials, and densities that can be used for stretching, strengthening, balance training, stability training, and self-massage.

**gait cycle:** The rhythmic alternating movements of the legs that result in the forward movement of the body, or the way we run or walk.

**hamstrings:** The three muscles of the posterior thigh (the semitendinosus, semimembranosus, and biceps femoris) that work to flex the knee and extend the hip.

**hand weight:** Any of a range of free weights that are often used in weight training and toning. Small hand weights are usually cast iron formed in the shape of a dumbbell, sometimes coated with rubber or neoprene for comfort.

**iliotibial band (ITB):** A thick band of fibrous tissue that runs down the outside of the leg, beginning at the hip and extending to the outer side of the tibia just below the knee joint. The band functions in concert with several of the thigh muscles to provide stability to the outside of the knee joint.

**lateral:** Located on, or extending toward, the outside.

**medial:** Located on, or extending toward, the middle.

**medicine ball:** A small weighted ball used in weight training and toning.

**neutral position (spine):** A spinal position resembling an S shape, consisting of an inward curve in the lower back, when viewed in profile.

**posterior:** Located behind.

**press:** An exercise movement that calls for moving a weight or other resistance away from the body.

**primary muscle:** One of the main muscles activated during a certain activity.

**pronation:** Turning inward. A pronated foot is one in which the heel bone angles inward and the arch tends to collapse. Opposite of *supination*.

**quadriceps:** A large muscle group (full name: quadriceps femoris) that includes the four prevailing muscles on the front of the thigh: the rectus femoris, vastus intermedius, vastus lateralis, and vastus medialis. It is the great extensor muscle of the knee, forming a large fleshy mass that covers the front and sides of the femur muscle.

**range of motion:** The distance and direction a joint can move between the flexed position and the extended position.

**resistance band:** Any rubber tubing or flat band device that provides a resistive force used for strength training. Also called a "fitness band," "Thera-Band," "Dyna-Band," "stretching band," and "exercise band."

**rotator muscle:** One of a group of muscles that assist the rotation of a joint, such as the hip or the shoulder.

**scapula:** The protrusion of bone on the mid to upper back, also known as the "shoulder blade."

**secondary muscle:** A muscle activated during a certain activity that usually works to support the primary muscles.

**squat:** An exercise movement that calls for moving the hips back and bending the knees and hips to lower the torso and an accompanying weight, and then returning to the upright position. A squat primarily targets the muscles of the thighs, hips, buttocks, and hamstrings.

**supination:** Turning outward. In running, supination is the insufficient inward roll of the foot after landing. This places extra stress on the foot and can result in iliotibial band syndrome, Achilles tendinitis or plantar fasciitis. Also known as "overpronation."

**Swiss ball:** A flexile, inflatable PVC ball measuring approximately 18 to 30 inches in circumference that is used for weight training, physical therapy, balance training and many other exercise regimens. It is also called a "balance ball," "fitness ball," "stability ball," "exercise ball," "gym ball," "physioball," "body ball," "therapy ball" and many other names.

**warm-up:** Any form of light exercise of short duration that prepares the body for more intense exercises.

**weight:** Refers to the plates or weight stacks, or the actual poundage listed on the bar or dumbbell.

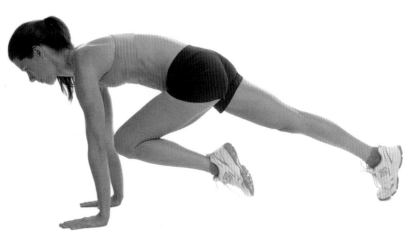

# GLOSSARY

## LATIN TERMS

*The following glossary explains the Latin scientific terminology used to describe the muscles of the human body. Certain words are derived from Greek, which is indicated in each instance.*

### CHEST

**coracobrachialis:** Greek *korakoeidés*, "ravenlike," and *brachium*, "arm"

**pectoralis (major and minor):** *pectus*, "breast"

### ABDOMEN

**obliquus externus:** *obliquus*, "slanting," and *externus*, "outward"

**obliquus internus:** *obliquus*, "slanting," and *internus*, "within"

**rectus abdominis:** *rego*, "straight, upright," and *abdomen*, "belly"

**serratus anterior:** *serra*, "saw," and *ante*, "before"

**transversus abdominis:** *transversus*, "athwart," and *abdomen*, "belly"

### NECK

**scalenus:** Greek *skalénós*, "unequal"

**semispinalis:** *semi*, "half," and *spinae*, "spine"

**splenius:** Greek *splénion*, "plaster, patch"

**sternocleidomastoideus:** Greek *stérnon*, "chest," Greek *kleís*, "key" and Greek *mastoeidés*, "breastlike"

### BACK

**erector spinae:** *erectus*, "straight," and *spina*, "thorn"

**latissimus dorsi:** *latus*, "wide," and *dorsum*, "back"

**multifidus spinae:** *multifid*, "to cut into divisions," and *spinae*, "spine"

**quadratus lumborum:** *quadratus*, "square, rectangular," and *lumbus*, "loin"

**rhomboideus:** Greek *rhembesthai*, "to spin"

**trapezius:** Greek *trapezion*, "small table"

### SHOULDERS

**deltoideus (anterior, medial, and posterior):** Greek *deltoeidés*, "delta-shaped"

**infraspinatus:** *infra*, "under," and *spina*, "thorn"

**levator scapulae:** *levare*, "to raise," and *scapulae*, "shoulder [blades]"

**subscapularis:** *sub*, "below," and *scapulae*, "shoulder [blades]"

**supraspinatus:** *supra*, "above," and *spina*, "thorn"

**teres (major and minor):** *teres*, "rounded"

### UPPER ARM

**biceps brachii:** *biceps*, "two-headed," and *brachium*, "arm"

**brachialis:** *brachium*, "arm"

**triceps brachii:** *triceps*, "three-headed" and *brachium*, "arm"

### LOWER ARM

**anconeus:** Greek *anconad*, "elbow"

**brachioradialis:** *brachium*, "arm," and *radius*, "spoke"

**extensor carpi radialis:** *extendere*, "to extend," Greek *karpós*, "wrist" and *radius*, "spoke"

**extensor digitorum:** *extendere*, "to extend," and *digitus*, "finger, toe"

**flexor carpi pollicis longus:** *flectere*, "to bend," Greek *karpós*, "wrist," *pollicis*, "thumb" and *longus*, "long"

**flexor carpi radialis:** *flectere*, "to bend," Greek *karpós*, "wrist" and *radius*, "spoke"

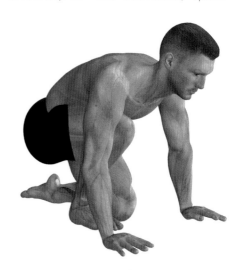

**flexor carpi ulnaris:** *flectere*, "to bend," Greek *karpós*, "wrist," and *ulnaris*, "forearm"

**flexor digitorum:** *flectere*, "to bend," and *digitus*, "finger, toe"

**palmaris longus:** *palmaris*, "palm," and *longus*, "long"

**pronator teres:** *pronate*, "to rotate," and *teres*, "rounded"

## HIPS

**gemellus (inferior and superior):** *geminus*, "twin"

**gluteus maximus:** Greek *gloutós*, "rump," and *maximus*, "largest"

**gluteus medius:** Greek *gloutós*, "rump" and *medialis*, "middle"

**gluteus minimus:** Greek *gloutós*, "rump" and *minimus*, "smallest"

**iliopsoas:** *ilium*, "groin," and Greek *psoa*, "groin muscle"

**iliacus:** *ilium*, "groin"

**obturator externus:** *obturare*, "to block" and *externus*, "outward"

**obturator internus:** *obturare*, "to block" and *internus*, "within"

**pectineus:** *pectin*, "comb"

**piriformis:** *pirum*, "pear," and *forma*, "shape"

**quadratus femoris:** *quadratus*, "square, rectangular," and *femur*, "thigh"

## UPPER LEG

**adductor longus:** *adducere*, "to contract," and *longus*, "long"

**adductor magnus:** *adducere*, "to contract," and *magnus*, "major"

**biceps femoris:** *biceps*, "two-headed," and *femur*, "thigh"

**gracilis:** *gracilis*, "slim, slender"

**rectus femoris:** *rego*, "straight, upright," and *femur*, "thigh"

**sartorius:** *sarcio*, "to patch" or "to repair"

**semimembranosus:** *semi*, "half," and *membrum*, "limb"

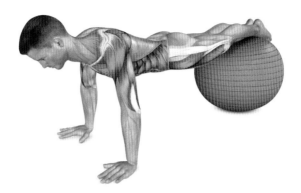

**semitendinosus:** *semi*, "half," and *tendo*, "tendon"

**tensor fasciae latae:** *tenere*, "to stretch," *fasciae*, "band," and *latae*, "laid down"

**vastus intermedius:** *vastus*, "immense, huge," and *intermedius*, "between"

**vastus lateralis:** *vastus*, "immense, huge," and lateralis, "side"

**vastus medialis:** *vastus*, "immense, huge," and *medialis*, "middle"

## LOWER LEG

**adductor digiti minimi:** *adducere*, "to contract," *digitus*, "finger, toe," and *minimum* "smallest"

**adductor hallucis:** *adducere*, "to contract," and *hallex*, "big toe"

**extensor digitorum longus:** *extendere*, "to extend," *digitus*, "finger, toe" and *longus*, "long"

**extensor hallucis longus:** *extendere*, "to extend," *hallex*, "big toe," and *longus*, "long"

**flexor digitorum longus:** *flectere*, "to bend," *digitus*, "finger, toe" and *longus*, "long"

**flexor hallucis longus:** *flectere*, "to bend," and *hallex*, "big toe" and *longus*, "long"

**gastrocnemius:** Greek *gastroknémía*, "calf [of the leg]"

**peroneus:** *peronei*, "of the fibula"

**plantaris:** *planta*, "the sole"

**soleus:** *solea*, "sandal"

**tibialis anterior:** *tibia*, "reed pipe," and *ante*, "before"

**tibialis posterior:** *tibia*, "reed pipe," and *posterus*, "coming after"

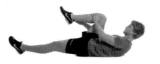

**Abdominal Kick**
pages 114–115

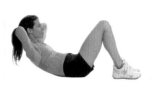

**Backward Ball Stretch**
pages 132–133

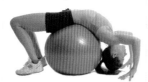

**Basic Crunch**
pages 110–111

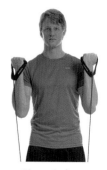

**Biceps Curl**
pages 134–135

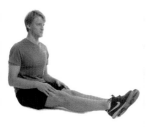

**Bilateral Seated Forward Bend**
pages 38–39

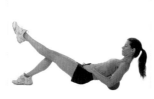

**Bridge with Leg Lift**
pages 122–123

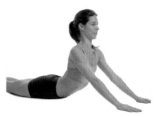

**Cobra Stretch**
pages 48–49

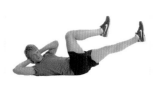

**Crossover Crunch**
pages 112–13

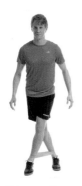

**Crossover Steps**
pages 74–75

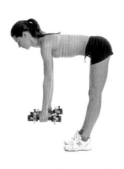

**Dumbbell Deadlift**
pages 66–67

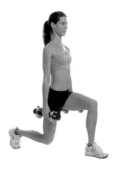

**Dumbbell Lunge**
pages 86–87

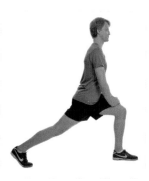

**Forward Lunge**
pages 28–29

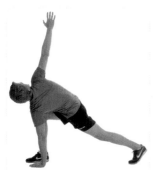

**Forward Lunge with Twist**
pages 30–31

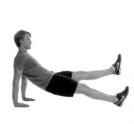

**Front Plank**
pages 106–107

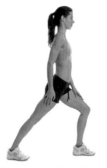

**Gastrocnemius Stretch**
page 58

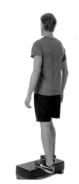

**Heel-Drop/Toe-Up Stretch**
pages 56–57

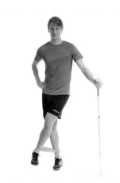

Hip Abduction and Adduction
pages 70–71

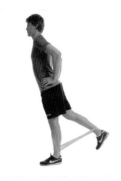

Hip Extension and Flexion
pages 68–69

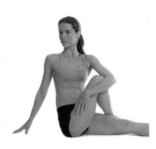

Hip/Iliotibial Band Stretch
pages 52–53

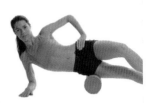

Iliotibial Band Release
pages 120–121

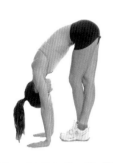

Iliotibial Band Stretch
page 60

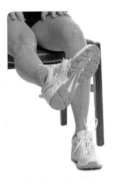

Knee Extension with Rotation
pages 88–89

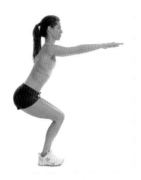

Knee Squat
pages 76–77

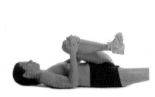

Knee-to-Chest Hug
pages 40–41

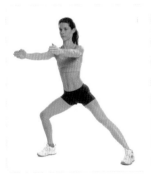

Lateral Low Lunge
pages 94–95

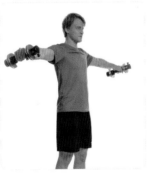

Lateral Shoulder Raise
pages 138–139

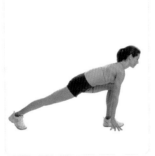

Low Lunge
pages 82–83

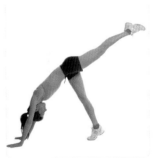

Plank Knee Pull-In
pages 116–117

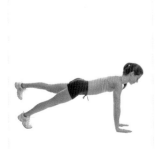

Plank Leg Extension
pages 80–81

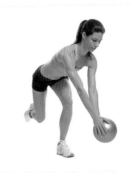

Power Squat
pages 98–99

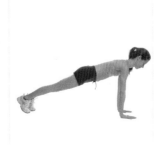

Push-Up
pages 124–125

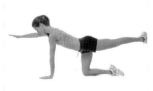

Quadruped Leg Lift
pages 104–105

# ICON INDEX

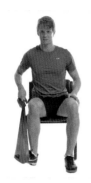

Resistance Band Ankle Stretches
pages 62–63

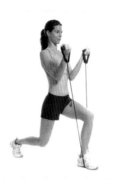

Resistance Band Lunge
pages 84–85

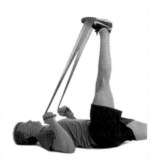

Resistance Band Tendon Stretch
page 61

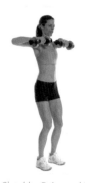

Shoulder Raise and Pull
pages 140–141

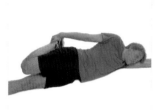

Side-Lying Knee Bend
pages 46–47

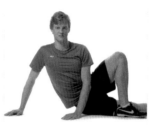

Side-Lying Rib Stretch
pages 50–51

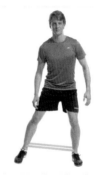

Side Steps
pages 72–73

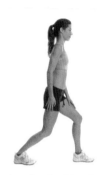

Soleus Stretch
page 59

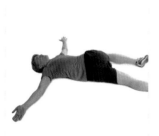

Spinal Rotation Stretch
pages 54–55

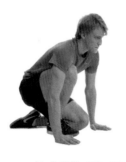

Sprinter Stretch
page 27

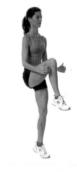

Standing Knee Crunch
pages 118–119

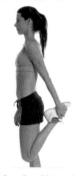

Standing Quadriceps Stretch
page 26

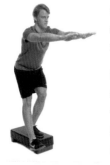

Step-Down
pages 96–97

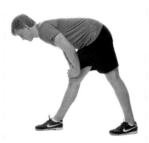

Straight-Leg Lunge
pages 32–33

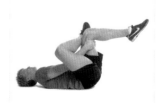

Supine Figure 4
pages 44–45

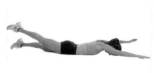

Swimming
pages 108–109

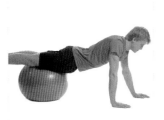

Swiss Ball Extension
pages 130–131

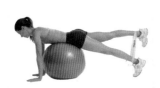

Swiss Ball Loop Extension
pages 78–79

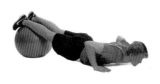

Swiss Ball Push-Up
pages 126–127

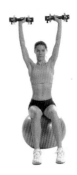

Swiss Ball Shoulder Press
page 136

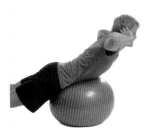

Swiss Ball Walkout
pages 128–129

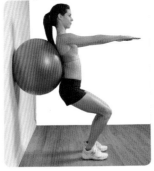

Swiss Ball Wall Sit
pages 92–93

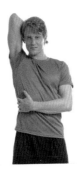

Triceps Extension
page 137

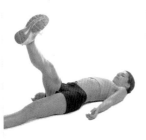

Unilateral Leg Circles
pages 102–103

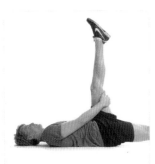

Unilateral Leg Raise
pages 42–43

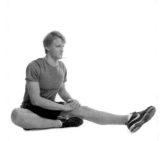

Unilateral Seated Forward Bend
pages 36–37

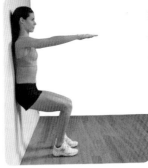

Wall Sit
pages 90–91

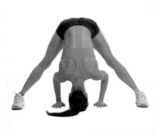

Wide-Legged Forward Bend
pages 34–35

# CREDITS & ACKNOWLEDGMENTS

All photographs by Jonathan Conklin/Jonathan Conklin Photography, Inc., except the following: pages 11 lightpoet/Shutterstock.com; 12 top Maridav/ Shutterstock.com; 12 bottom Gerald Bernard/Shutterstock.com; 12 left picamaniac/ Shutterstock.com; 14 Maridav/Shutterstock.com; 15 xc/Shutterstock.com; 16 PeterG/ Shutterstock.com; 17 Warren Goldswain/Shutterstock.com; 19 bottom left Maridav/ Shutterstock.com; 20 Marc Dietrich/Shutterstock.com

Models: Sara Blowers and Nicolay Alexandrov

All large anatomical illustrations by Hector Aiza/3D Labz Animation India (www.3dlabz.com), with small insets by Linda Bucklin/Shutterstock.com, pages 18 and 19 top right by Alila Sao Mai/Shutterstock.com, and page 21 top and bottom by design36/Shutterstock.com

## Acknowledgments

I want to take this opportunity to thank my parents, Drs. Philip and Theresa Striano, for guiding me through the years to get to this point in my life. Dad, although my time with you was short, your sacrifice and conviction for your profession, patients, and family will always be a guiding force for me. I also want to acknowledge my three sisters, Terri, Thomasina, and Tara, for the their love and support.

Dale Daniel for your hard work and keeping my doors open.

My t⋯ ⋯th joy, pride, and
chal⋯ ⋯Stacy, thank you both
for t⋯

I firr⋯ ⋯their interpersonal
inte⋯ ⋯eople, who throughout
my⋯ ⋯hool, the Stern, Allen,
Kho⋯ ⋯n and Marshall football
and⋯ ⋯ers, Pilzers, Smiths,
No⋯

In l⋯ ⋯passion of running and
exe⋯

Tha⋯ ⋯e.

The⋯ ⋯olved in the creation
of t⋯ ⋯anager Karen Prince,
pro⋯ ⋯dam Moore; designer
Ter⋯